SELF-HARM IN YOUNG PEOPLE

A Therapeutic Assessment Manual

T0187913

Dr Dennis Ougrin MBBS MRCPsych,
Kraupl Taylor Research Fellow,
Institute of Psychiatry,
London, UK

Dr Tobias Zundel MBBS MRCPsych,
Tavistock and Portman NHS Foundation Trust,
London, UK

Dr Audrey V. Ng MBBCh MRCPsych MA,
Central and North West London NHS Foundation Trust,
London, UK

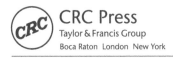

CRC Press
Taylor & Francis Group
Boca Raton London New York

CRC Press is an imprint of the
Taylor & Francis Group, an **informa** business

CRC Press
Taylor & Francis Group
6000 Broken Sound Parkway NW, Suite 300
Boca Raton, FL 33487-2742

© 2009 by Taylor & Francis Group, LLC
CRC Press is an imprint of Taylor & Francis Group, an Informa business

No claim to original U.S. Government works

Printed in the United States of America on acid-free paper
Version Date: 20121026

International Standard Book Number: 978-0-340-98726-1 (Paperback)

Visit the Taylor & Francis Web site at
http://www.taylorandfrancis.com

and the CRC Press Web site at
http://www.crcpress.com

Contents

Foreword

The full extent of self-harm in adolescents is becoming increasingly apparent. Recent studies in the United Kingdom which have used a fairly tight definition of self-harm have shown that as many as one in ten 15 and 16 year-olds have a history of self-harm, most having self-harmed in the previous year. Studies using essentially the same methodology have shown similar findings for several other European countries and Australia. Surveys using more varied methods in some other countries have suggested an even greater prevalence of self-harm. All such studies have consistently shown self-harm to be far more common in girls than boys. While many adolescents who self-harm may not come to the attention of clinicians, at least initially, studies based on presentations to accident and emergency departments of general hospitals have, since the 1970s, consistently shown self-harm to be extremely common and indeed one of the most frequent reasons for general hospital presentation by young people.

Self-harm in adolescents usually indicates significant psychological distress, which amounts to psychiatric disorder in many individuals. Therefore the extent of the problem is indicative of considerable levels of unhappiness in adolescents, which general population surveys have shown to have increased over time, especially in girls. Unsurprisingly, self-harm by a young person usually has major effects on other family members and friends. The large number of adolescents presenting to hospitals following self-harm puts considerable demands on accident and emergency, general medical and psychiatric services. Self-harm is also a significant issue in schools.

It is not surprising therefore that attention is increasingly being paid to prevention of self-harm and treatment of those who have self-harmed. This need is highlighted by longitudinal studies, which have shown that in a significant proportion of cases self-harm may have significant implications for future adjustment in young adulthood, not just in terms of risk of continued self-harm but also for other mental health and social outcomes. While measures to help prevent self-harm in adolescents are essential, there is a major need for effective care for adolescents who have self-harmed. More attention is therefore being paid to therapeutic initiatives. This book represents such an initiative.

What makes this book so special is that, following a clear presentation of what is known about the nature and causes of self-harm, Dennis Ougrin and his colleagues focus in great detail on assessment and initial treatment of adolescents who have self-harmed. The authors have clearly thought very carefully about these aspects of care. In particular they have developed original ideas about how to make the assessment of adolescents who have self-harmed more effective, rightly labelling their approach 'therapeutic assessment'. They have shown that such an approach may enhance engagement with subsequent therapy. It is widely recognised that levels of attendance for treatment are often extremely low in adolescents offered aftercare following self-harm. While family and other external factors may play a role in this, how useful or indeed appropriate the individual adolescent thinks such care is likely to be will be strongly influenced by his or her interactions with a clinician at the initial assessment. Unless willingness to attend for therapy is enhanced only a minority of individuals will receive aftercare. Even those adolescents who do not go on to have further treatment are likely to benefit from a therapeutic assessment. In producing this book, which in large part is a manual of how to do it, the authors have therefore done a great service to clinicians working with adolescents who have self-harmed. In designing their assessment and treatment approaches they have drawn on elements of various types of psychological therapeutics. They have also clearly responded to feedback from young people themselves. Their extensive use of diagrams as part of the assessment and therapeutic process will make their approach especially appealing to both adolescents themselves and to clinicians.

This book will be of value and considerable interest to clinicians of all professional backgrounds who are in a position to provide help to young people with thoughts of self-harm or suicide, and especially those who have carried out acts of self-harm. Clinicians will find their skills and sense of competence greatly increased by reading this book. The most important outcome is that this is likely to result in more young people benefiting from assessment and hence engaging in treatment, and therefore having an enhanced chance of a positive long-term outcome.

Professor Keith Hawton
Director, Centre for Suicide Research
University of Oxford
Oxford, UK

Preface

The idea of Therapeutic Assessment was conceived several years ago when I was a second-year trainee psychiatrist assessing a young person while on call (I'll call her Meg). She presented to an inner-city hospital emergency department following a massive overdose and her life was in severe danger. I saw Meg after she was medically "cleared", that is to say her physical health was stable. The psychiatric history was very difficult to take – Meg had experienced multiple traumas and could not speak about them because of the unmanageable feelings her story was likely to evoke. At one stage she started crying uncontrollably and it took me a long time to soothe her. On the basis of what little information was available, I gradually started to form the view that Meg was suffering from severe depression.

At the time I was studying the principles of several psychological therapies. It was obvious, however, that the techniques I was learning were geared towards longer-term treatment and I felt powerless in the face of an acute crisis. Meg was admitted to a psychiatric unit under a section of the Mental Health Act – she had very negative memories of a previous admission but the risk of suicide seemed overwhelming. When I came to say goodbye, she was crying and told me I was another person who had made her go through "this hell" again.

Several ideas emerged from this experience. Firstly, it was clear that self-harm presentation represents a crisis but also a time of therapeutic opportunity – except the therapeutic opportunity is frequently missed. Secondly, the process of self-harm assessment might well be an alienating rather than a therapeutic experience for many young people. The assessment may sometimes be little more than a clinician asking a young person lots of difficult questions in order to make up his or her mind whether the young person is safe to go home or not. The questions may of course increase levels of distress, which the assessor then may not know how to handle adequately. Thirdly, it seemed obvious that even if some kind of therapeutic intervention was used, it was unlikely that a single technique would work with all young people. Finally, it was also clear that no matter how effective our interventions for managing self-harming behaviour are or will become in the future, they are all pretty much useless unless we can engage young people in the therapeutic process.

Therapeutic Assessment is an attempt to address, to a degree, these problems. Its main tenets are as follows. Firstly, a therapeutic intervention at the time of distress, compared to standard psychosocial history and risk assessment, appears to improve young people's satisfaction and their willingness to engage with further therapeutic work. Secondly, Therapeutic Assessment draws on a vast range of evidence-based interventions to create a therapeutic "toolkit" that individual practitioners can use. Thirdly, Therapeutic Assessment is simple and easy to learn and is designed for use by all mental health professionals who assess young people following an episode of self-harm.

This book consists of two parts. Part I is called "The Framework" and Part II is called "The Tools".

Part I is about facts – the building blocks of the framework Therapeutic Assessment is based on. There are three key questions addressed in Part I: 1."What is self-harm?" 2. "What are the key facts about self-harm?" 3. "What is the rationale for Therapeutic Assessment?"

Part II is about tools – the building blocks of Therapeutic Assessment practice. There are three key questions addressed in Part II: 1. "How to help patients understand self-harm?" 2. "How to motivate and instil hope?" 3. "How to explore alternatives to self-harm?" Therapeutic Assessment provides clinicians with a set of tools to achieve these goals.

The readers of this manual may well already be using a form of assessment that has some therapeutic elements. The authors of this manual would not claim that the techniques described here are necessarily better than whatever techniques work for individual, experienced practitioners. Moreover, if these techniques were evidence based we would like to incorporate them into the future development of Therapeutic Assessment. There is no limit to the number of tools in the TA "toolkit" and we hope that even the most experienced therapists may find some of the ideas useful.

On behalf of the authors,
Dennis Ougrin

Acknowledgements

Above all I would like to thank my wife Oksana and daughter Anastasia. This manual would not have been possible without you.

Special thanks go to the patients and the clinicians of the South London and Maudsley NHS Foundation Trust for their decisive contribution to the development of Therapeutic Assessment.

I am indebted and grateful to the following people and organisations who made this manual possible: Partha Banerjea, Bruce Clark, Jo Fletcher, Peter Hindley, Gordana Milavic, KAH Mirza, Mark Perry, Richard Corrigall and Mima Simic for facilitating the clinical application of Therapeutic Assessment; Derek Bolton, Robert Goodman, Keith Hawton, Eric Taylor and Emily Simonoff for academic supervision; Sophie Browning, Evan George, Tony Ryle, Amrit Sacha, Patrick Smith and Troy Tranah for psychotherapy advice.

Finally, I'd like to thank the South London and Maudsley NHS Foundation Trust Charitable Funds (Chairman Kumar Jacob) and the Psychiatric Research Trust (Chairman David Goldberg) for their support and for the inspiring and selfless work they do in facilitating research and innovation.

Dennis Ougrin

I wish to express my debt to all the young people I have had the privilege of meeting during the work of developing and establishing Therapeutic Assessment as an approach towards better serving their needs.

I would like to thank my family, particularly my daughters Noa and Uma, for their continuous support and inspiration, Melissa Greer and all the friends who have been there over recent years.

I also acknowledge my gratitude to colleagues both past and present who have encouraged and guided me over the years. I would like to specifically mention Peter Loader, who introduced me to child and adolescent psychiatry, Rob Senior, Mark Berelowitz for supporting the research work at the Royal Free Hospital, my fellow SpRs at the Tavistock Centre and Dennis Ougrin.

Tobias Zundel

To all the patients who have inspired me, both young and old, and my mentors who have guided me, my gratitude. To my husband, Dr Triet Hoang and my little sunshine Zac without whose patience and support I would never have done this, my love. Finally to the people who read this book and those they try to help, my hopes.

Audrey Ng

Additional contributors

Dr Colin Campbell BSc MBChB MRCPsych
Honorary Consultant Forensic Psychiatrist,
South London and Maudsley NHS Foundation Trust,
London, UK

Dr Elaine Chung MBBS MRCPsych
Consultant Child and Adolescent Psychiatrist,
Royal Free Hospital NHS Trust,
London, UK

Dr Saqib Latif
Speciality Registrar in Child and Adolescent Psychiatry,
South London and Maudsley NHS Foundation Trust,
London, UK

Dr Marinos Kyriakopoulos MBBS MRCPsych
Consultant Child and Adolescent Psychiatrist,
South London and Maudsley NHS Foundation Trust,
London, UK

Dr Matthias Schwannauer MA DPsych PhD CPsychol AFBPsS
Senior Lecturer in Child and Adolescent Clinical Psychology,
University of Edinburgh,
Edinburgh, UK

Dr Paul Wilkinson MRCPsych MD
Clinical Lecturer and Locum Consultant in Child and Adolescent Psychiatry and Interpersonal Psychotherapist,
University of Cambridge,
Cambridge, UK

CHAPTER 1

DEFINING SELF-HARM

Dennis Ougrin
Tobias Zundel

Introduction

Readers might be surprised to find a whole chapter dedicated to the definition of self-harm at the very beginning of this book. It may be even more surprising to know that in many ways this chapter is not comprehensive and certain aspects of the discussion around defining self-harm will be developed further in subsequent chapters. The authors' decision to write this chapter was based on the assumption that without a clear definition it is impossible to interpret any literature on self-harm, including this book. 'What do the authors mean when they say self-harm?' should probably be the first question readers ask themselves when reading any material on the subject.

It may be that the readers of this book have already crystallised their own definitions of self-harm. We suspect, however, that for many this is not the case. While it is not suggested that readers necessarily accept the definition presented here, for operational purposes it is important to bear it in mind while reading the rest of this book.

The historical divide in defining self-harm

Self-harm as a form of human behaviour has attracted considerable research attention in the last 20 years,[1] but it has existed for millennia, perhaps for as long as humans existed, in different cultures and in different geographical areas.[2] It was described variably in the Bible as a sign of madness, a deed of the devil or a way to salvation (Mark 9: 47–8, Kings 18: 28, Mark 5: 5, Matthew 6: 22–3).[3] Differences in the underlying motivation and intent were at the heart of the understanding of self-harm. It will not surprise readers that, as with many other ancient debates, this one has not been resolved to date. The history of modern self-harm definitions is also fraught with disputes. These still revolve primarily around its meaning.

One of the first attempts to introduce sub-categorisation to suicide-related behaviour dates back to 1938, when Meninger[4] attempted to sub-categorise self-mutilative behaviour. In 1964 Stengel[5] proposed that people who committed suicide and suicide attempters represented two distinct populations. However, according to Stengel, strictly speaking, a 'true' suicide attempt should refer only to those who failed to die after having tried to kill themselves. Many authorities disagreed with this nomenclature, especially feminist writers who suggested the more inclusive term of 'suicidal behaviour'.[6,7] A driver for this change was a suggestion that men were perceived more competent in completing suicide whereas women were seen as failing.

Kreitman's seminal work on parasuicide[8] was designed to produce a broad category of suicide-related behaviours and has been widely used in Europe[9-11] and in the USA[12] until recently. Many contemporary definitions of suicidal behaviour are based on this concept.

The American perspective, epitomised by the early work of Beck and colleagues,[13,14] placed classification of intent at the foundation of suicidal behaviour classification and argued that suicidal behaviour should be defined, researched and treated differently depending on the presence or the absence of the intent to die.

For the last 50 years the field of self-harm has been divided between those experts who consider self-harm to be a broad continuum of self-injurious behaviours, irrespective of intent, and those who argue in favour of firm categorisation of self-harm into that with and without suicidal intent.

In the remainder of this chapter the authors will focus on these two conceptual nomenclatures broadly representing American and European/Australasian approaches, which will somewhat arbitrarily be called the Beck–O'Carroll–Silverman nomenclature and the Kreitman–Hawton–De Leo nomenclature.

Nomenclature and classification of self-harm

Although the terms 'nomenclature' and 'classification' have some overlap, they are distinct. Nomenclature seeks to define the basic concepts and is concerned with terminology and definitions, whereas classification seeks to comprehensibly describe the phenomena. A classification system is impossible without clear nomenclature. Nomenclature of self-harm is confusing and many authorities use self-harm terminology to denote different concepts. The field is probably still at the point of developing nomenclature rather than classification.[15] Some of the difficulties with establishing self-harm nomenclature are considered below.

The basis of self-harm nomenclature: looking for objective measures

All self-harm nomenclatures are based on the following four concepts: intent, method, outcome and lethality.

Outcome of self-harm is probably the most objective and non-controversial domain. Method of self-harm is somewhat more difficult to establish with confidence as it is largely based on self-reporting. Method and outcome are closely linked and it might be possible to verify both with an examination and/or investigations. Epidemiological studies rely primarily on subjective self-report when establishing the method of self-harm.[16,17]

Lethality can be misleading as an indicator of the severity of self-harm. This is primarily due to a variable gap between objective and subjective lethality.

Intent is the most controversial dimension of the four and the least amenable to objective evaluation. In essence, authorities are split on the role of intent in self-harm nomenclature. Both European and American nomenclatures use the concept of intent, but in different ways. Whereas the Beck–O'Carroll–Silverman nomenclature uses intent to differentiate between suicidal and non-suicidal self-harm, the Kreitman–Hawton–De Leo approach argues that intent cannot be used as a reliable differentiator and all non-fatal self-harm may or may not be underpinned by suicidal intent. A further disagreement exists about the taxonomy of suicidal thinking. American nomenclatures usually include suicidal thinking in the spectrum of 'suicidality'. European nomenclatures consider behaviour separately from thoughts.

What is intent?

According to the Merriam Webster dictionary, intent (intention) can be defined as the determination to act in a certain way.[18] It refers to the aim of an action, although the action itself is not required.[19] Motivation (motives, reasons) is a driving force underpinning intent; for example, a wish to escape, desire to obtain relief, to end suffering, etc.[20] Motivation and intent are sometimes confused in the literature[21] and it is intent rather than motivation that is used as a basis for self-harm nomenclature.

Intent: explicit versus implicit

Like lethality, intent can be thought about as subjective and objective,[14] although this distinction is not made universally. A rather controversial approach to intent was formalised in O'Carroll's nomenclature, dichotomising 'zero' versus 'non-zero' intent.[22] Posner et al.[23] followed this logic, recognising further that 'non-zero' intent could be substantiated by either an explicit subjective report or inferred from the subject's behaviour. Rudd[24] further argues that the assessment of objective evidence of intent is more important than the subjective report. Brent et al.[25] see suicidal intent as consisting of four orthogonal factors:

- belief about intent
- preparation before attempt
- prevention of discovery
- communication.

These four factors vary in the degree to which they can be assessed objectively.

Finally, while recognising the importance of intent, other authors argue that the distinction between subjective and objective intent may be hard to interpret.[26]

Intent: importance

Although there is disagreement among researchers about the role of suicidal intent in the definition of self-harm, most authorities have come to the conclusion that it is an important aspect of risk assessment.[10,27,28] Subjects with a combination of suicidal and non-suicidal self-harm may score higher on several measures of psychopathology and risk-taking behaviour.[29]

Intent: measurement reliability

Beck and colleagues[13,14,30] argue that measuring suicidal intent is essential for both clinical and research reasons and can be done reliably. In recent reports, Beck's group have moved to a more dialectical view of suicidal intent, balancing the wish to live and the wish to die and replicating the previous work of Kovacs and Beck.[31,32]

The authors who consider intent hard to measure reliably, do so on the basis of the following arguments: that intent is frequently assessed incorrectly and/or is subject to recall bias; that many subjects are unclear about their intent; that suicidal and non-suicidal intent may coexist and both suicidal and non-suicidal behaviour frequently occur within the same individual.

Freeman et al.[33] showed that a vast majority of so-called suicide attempts are in fact episodes of self-injury without suicidal intent. The authors proposed to eliminate the term suicide attempt and replace it with the term self-harm irrespective of intent. A similar question was raised by Meehan et al.,[34] who found that for every 10 reported suicide attempts only one required hospitalisation. This, the authors concluded, suggests that the term is overused and an independent verification is needed for an accurate classification of suicide attempts.

Subjects often present a variety of reasons for self-harm and frequently different reasons coexist.[9,35] Common overlapping reasons for self-harm include the following: to die, to escape from unbearable circumstances, to influence others and to feel better.

Finally, in the studies of non-suicidal self-harmers a significant proportion of subjects report suicidal as well as non-suicidal self-harm.[36,37]

Intent: assessment

Bearing in mind the theoretical differences outlined above, it should be no surprise that measuring intent presents researchers and clinicians with difficulties. The issue of assessing intent is also a complex one. Beck and colleagues[13,14,30] argue that measuring suicidal intent is essential for both clinical and research reasons and can be done reliably.

Following on from his ideas on self-harm classification, Beck et al.[14] created the Suicide Intent Scale that incorporated both objective and subjective factors designed to measure suicidal intent. Although this instrument undoubtedly represented a breakthrough in the area of the assessment of a suicidal person, it did not resolve the fundamental question of the role that intent plays in self-harm nomenclature.

Posner et al.[23] recently developed the Columbia Classification Algorithm of Suicide Assessment (C-CASA), a diagnostic schedule designed to arrive at a differentiation between suicidal and non-suicidal self-harm. The measure includes an important category of indeterminate or potentially suicidal events where suicidal intent is unknown. The impact of this instrument remains to be seen, although a significant advantage of the C-CASA is that it recognises difficulties in classifying the presence or otherwise of suicidal intent in many cases.

What is lethality?

Subjective and objective lethality are both important in the assessment of risk and are discussed in the nomenclature of self-harm. Typically, lethality refers to the medical or biological danger to life.[38] As applied to the assessment of risk of death by suicide, lethality specifically refers to the dangerousness inherent in the suicidal act. It reflects the potential for death associated with the means used to attempt suicide.[39] From this perspective, firearms, jumping from heights or in front of a train, hanging, suffocation, asphyxiation by carbon monoxide, and drowning may be considered high-lethality methods, whereas wrist cutting, some drug overdoses and poisonings may be considered low-lethality methods.

There is a recognised association between objective lethality and risk of dying by suicide.[25] Other authors failed to find an independent association between objective lethality and risk of further episodes of self-harm,[40] although it was strongly associated with intent. Even those subjects presenting with near-fatal self-harm report no suicidal intent in about a third of cases.[41]

Brown et al.[27] found a minimal association between the degree of suicide intent and the extent of medical lethality for patients who attempted suicide, suggesting that suicidal intent and lethality are independent dimensions of suicidal behaviour. Both characteristics, however, were related to subsequent risk. In that study over half of the attempters had inaccurate expectations of medical lethality. These results reconfirmed the previous finding[13] that a low correlation between intent and objective lethality could be moderated by subjective lethality. On the basis of the authors' arguments, subjective lethality is thought to be a better predictor of risk than objective lethality. On the other hand, objective lethality, being linked with outcome, provides a better basis for nomenclature.

There is no self-harm nomenclature developed purely on the basis of self-harm lethality at present. In a review, Skegg[42] proposed the principles for such a nomenclature, but this nomenclature cannot be considered comprehensive at present.

The spectrum ranges from highly lethal behaviours like shooting and hanging at one extreme to cutting and burning at the other extreme.

Most modern tools of lethality assessment use both objective and subjective lethality items.[43]

What are outcome and method?

Method and outcome of self-harm are at the heart of all known nomenclatures.

Method refers to the way or the process that is used by the subject to self-harm, which then leads to one of three possible outcomes: death, survival with injuries or survival without injuries.

People who self-harm employ a great variety of methods and could switch from one method to another. The method may be related to the lethality of the act, although many young people may over or underestimate the lethality of their chosen method of self-harm.[44]

The method of self-harm is often used as a way of defining a research population[45-47] as it avoids the problems associated with the definitions that rely on more subjective measures. De Leo *et al.*[48] argue that on their own, outcome and methods could not be regarded as sufficient factors for establishing a self-harm nomenclature although they are necessary components.

What are the leading self-harm nomenclatures available?

Beck–O'Carroll–Silverman

An attempt by O'Carroll *et al.*[22] to create a universal nomenclature was underpinned by the efforts of the National Institute of Mental Health and the American Association of Suicidology. The nomenclature working group was formed to clarify the nomenclature used in the field to describe suicidal ideations and suicidal behaviours. It followed Beck's ideas on nomenclature of self-harm,[22] although Beck is one of the authors of a separate nomenclature.[49]

The Beck–O'Carroll–Silverman nomenclature appeared to recognise that suicide-related behaviours could be subdivided into two main groups: instrumental suicide-related behaviour (with no intent to die) and suicidal acts (with intent to die). The nomenclature was not adopted universally[19] and a revision was attempted recently.[50] One of the principal difficulties, as always, proved to be the assessment of suicidal intent. In the original nomenclature O'Carroll *et al.* discussed the concept of 'zero intent to die' versus 'non-zero intent to die'. The concept of non-zero intent to die came under criticism as being too broad and not taking into account the difficulties of assessing intent in many patients.[19]

In a revision of O'Carroll's nomenclature Silverman et al.[50] proposed a different way forward, perhaps bridging to some degree the controversy surrounding the issue of suicidal intent. Having rejected the dichotomous approach to the definition of intent, these authors proposed that intent may be present, absent or undetermined and subjects could have sustained no injuries, some injuries or died as a result of their behaviour.

Silverman et al.[50] specifically took into account the European view that self-harm could be defined irrespective of the intent. This attempt at bridging the differences is to be welcomed. The authors took into account the fact that in recent years the word 'deliberate' was dropped in the previously ubiquitous term 'deliberate self-harm' by many European researchers following a representation of service users to the Royal College of Psychiatrists.[28] The term 'self-harm' was subsequently also adopted by the National Institute for Health and Clinical Excellence (NICE) in the UK.[51]

Silverman et al.'s nomenclature is not, however, devoid of problems. First, it does not take into account the issue of lethality – one of the key defining characteristics of suicide-related behaviour. Second, it does not fully take into account the issue of the suicide-related communication and thinking, without suicidal intent. Thus, if the logic of the nomenclature is to be followed, a suicide-related communication and plan should not be called 'suicide threat type 1' or 'suicide plan type 1' (type 1 indicates absence of suicide intent) but rather self-harm threat or plan type 1.

Kreitman–Hawton–De Leo

Hawton et al.[16] define (deliberate) self-harm as intentional self-injury or self-poisoning, irrespective of type of motivation or degree of suicidal intent. This approach is linked to Kreitman's original definition of parasuicide. Many European investigators use this definition[11] and it is also used in Australia[52] and New Zealand.[53]

De Leo et al.[48] proposed a nomenclature that recognised the importance of intent but did not place it at the centre of self-harm definition. These authors described the evolution of the self-harm nomenclature during the WHO/EURO study on parasuicide. The initial definition adopted by the study was as follows:[48]

> *Parasuicide is an act with a nonfatal outcome in which an individual deliberately initiates a non-habitual behaviour that, without intervention from others, will cause self-harm, or deliberately ingests a substance in excess of the prescribed or generally recognized therapeutic dosage, and which is aimed at realizing changes which the subject desired, via the actual or expected physical consequences.*

This definition did not distinguish between behaviour aimed at suicide or otherwise and was closest to the definition of self-harm currently in use in the UK. Parasuicide and attempted suicide were used interchangeably, recognising the difficulties inherent in ascertaining intent. Furthermore, the authors initially recognised Kreitman's suggestion that using terms such as deliberate self-harm, self-injury or self-poisoning tends to obfuscate the relationship between these behaviours and suicide[8]. A few years later, in 1999, the group embraced an outcome-based orientation to the definitions, proposing the use of the terms 'fatal' and 'nonfatal' suicidal behaviour.[48] The study itself was renamed the WHO/EURO Multicenter Study on Suicidal Behaviour. Non-fatal suicidal behaviour was then defined as a 'nonhabitual act with nonfatal outcome that the individual, expecting to, or taking the risk to die or to inflict bodily harm, initiated and carried out with the purpose of bringing about wanted changes'. The proposed nomenclature then appeared to agree that non-fatal suicidal behaviour may have no suicidal intent or suicidal intent that is greater than zero. Although the intent was recognised as important, the nomenclature clearly indicated that non-fatal suicidal behaviour may or may not be underpinned by intent to die. The importance of this nomenclature is in its attempt to bridge the differences among research groups. These authors also recognised that even collaborators of the same big trial may disagree and may change their definitions over time.

The Kreitman–Hawton–De Leo nomenclature has several limitations. First, it focuses specifically on self-harm as a behaviour and does not include suicidal/self-harm thinking and planning. Second, the nomenclature is based on the premise that self-harm behaviour must be intentional; however, its lethality and suicidal intent are disregarded.

This brief overview precludes a full discussion of the available nomenclatures. The examples discussed are chosen primarily to illustrate the nature of the debate and the way different researchers think about self-harm. Although the two approaches described differ with respect to the role of suicidal intent in the definition of self-harm, it is worth noting that the latest papers appear to use more consensual language, recognising on one hand the importance of intent for the definition of self-harm and on the other hand acknowledging potential pitfalls in its assessment.

Could self-harm be categorised on the basis of intent?

We have already discussed the controversy surrounding the measurement of intent. There is no current agreement whether or not intent can be measured reliably. But could there be other characteristics that could reliably distinguish between the two groups? This discussion can only make sense when looking at the two extremes of the spectrum, i.e. people with categorically no intent to die and people who have definite intent to die. Most researchers, however, agree that there is a large group of subjects in whom intent cannot be assessed with any degree of certainty. In addition, there are many subjects who display both suicidal and non-suicidal self-harm at different times. The following discussion will focus on the question of whether or not suicidal and non-suicidal self-harm meet criteria for separate disorders.

Would suicidal and non-suicidal self-harm meet St Louis criteria for a separate disorder?

Feighner et al.[54] propose that diagnostic validity of a psychiatric disorder relies on the following five factors (known as the St Louis criteria):

1. clinical description
2. laboratory studies
3. specific exclusion criteria for other disorders
4. follow-up outcome
5. genetic (family) studies.

Clinical description

It is proposed that a non-suicidal and suicidal self-harming individual could be differentiated on the basis of the following characteristics: intent, lethality, method, repetition/chronicity and psychological characteristics (constriction of cognition, level of psychological pain, severity of hopelessness and other depressive symptoms or emotions in the aftermath).[55] Most of the proposed differences have not been demonstrated in large population-based studies directly comparing suicidal versus non-suicidal groups.

Some of the difficulties associated with the use of lethality and intent to differentiate the two groups were discussed above. Although in many cases intent is difficult to establish, some subjects are clear that when they self-harm they do not want to die, that their aim is to modify rather than to terminate consciousness and that they tend to feel better after an episode of self-harm.[1,55-57] There are well-documented differences between the risk implications of low versus high suicide intent in self-harm;[28,58] however, the authors who showed these differences did not distinguish between no-intent and high-intent populations.

Differences in observed behaviour

There are several studies proposing that those who self-harm without suicidal intent are more likely to use low-lethality methods as opposed to high-lethality in suicide attempters.[36,59] No method of self-harm, however, is exclusively related to suicidal intent. Furthermore, subjects may use different methods of self-harm at different times.[37] Up to 70 per cent of subjects who self-harm without suicidal intent also attempt suicide.[37] Guertin et al.[29] view non-suicidal self-harm as a complicating factor in suicidal self-harm. In this study the subjects who engaged in non-suicidal self-harm (referred to as self-mutilative behaviour, SMB) as well as suicidal self-harm were significantly more likely to be diagnosed with oppositional defiant disorder, major depression and dysthymia, and had higher scores on measures of hopelessness, loneliness, anger, risk taking, reckless behaviour and alcohol use than did suicide attempters without SMB.

An example of an association between self-harm and suicide was tragically demonstrated by Vincent van Gogh, who cut off a part of his ear in 1888 before eventually dying by suicide.

Regarding chronicity, again there are studies indicating that the subjects who self-harm with no suicidal intent are more likely to engage in repetitive self-harming behaviour[56]. However, an important minority of subjects who repeatedly attempt suicide has also been described.[60] Up to 55 per cent of subjects with non-suicidal self-injury also repeatedly attempt suicide.[37]

Differences in sociodemographic characteristics, prevalence and onset

Non-sucidal self-harm may be more common and increasing,[61,62] whereas suicidal self-harm may be less prevalent and falling.[63] However, this conclusion cannot be reached with confidence because of the methodological problems of the prevalence studies and the absence of adequate head-to-head comparisons.

There are very few studies directly comparing sociodemographic characteristics of suicide attempters versus non-suicidal self-harmers.[37,55,57,64] The largest study investigating these differences found a preponderance of females among the suicidal self-harmers, lower educational attainment in the suicidal group and a higher prevalence of non-suicidal self-harm in the northern and eastern USA versus southern and western USA.[17] The study design was not ideal. The sample was drawn from young people who all initially classified their behaviour as suicidal; however, nearly half of those were subsequently reclassified as having carried out a 'suicidal gesture', i.e. self-harm without true suicidal intent.

There are suggestions that non-suicidal self-harm is equally prevalent among males and females,[61,65] although other studies found a female preponderance.[66] Other possible sociodemographic differences may include a higher prevalence of non-suicidal self-harm in Caucasians.[61,62]

There are no consistent findings differentiating suicidal and non-suicidal behaviour in terms of time of onset. The frequency of both behaviours increases in adolescence and young adulthood and then diminishes over time.[67] However, there is a further peak in suicidal self-harm in later life, probably not mirrored by non-suicidal self-harm.

Differences in diagnostic correlates

Both suicidal and non-suicidal self-harmers overwhelmingly (in about 90 per cent of cases) satisfy diagnostic criteria for one or more psychiatric disorders,[37,38] depression being the most common diagnosis in both groups. These results, however, only apply to the clinical samples and it may be that in the non-referred adolescents the rate of psychiatric disorders is much lower. Nock and Kessler[17] also found that suicidal versus non-suicidal self-harmers have a higher prevalence of depression, drug abuse and drug dependence, conduct disorder and antisocial personality disorder, phobias and multiple diagnoses. The methodological problems of this study were discussed above, however the results are important in the light of other studies, finding differences between the two groups in depression scores, suicidal thinking, attitude to life and post-traumatic stress disorder.[61,68]

Other correlates

Adolescents engaging in non-suicidal versus suicidal self-harm may be more likely to have a history of sexual molestation and physical assault[17]. It may be that the relationship between sexual abuse and non-suicidal self-harm is mediated by dissociation.[69]

Problem-solving deficits in the subjects who attempt suicide are one of the most consistent findings in both the adult and the adolescent literature;[70,71] however, recent studies demonstrated similar deficits in non-suicidal samples.[72] It may be that adolescents with non-suicidal self-harm differ from suicidal samples on measures of thought suppression[73] and emotional reactivity,[74] but no direct comparisons are yet available.

In summary, there may be significant differences between adolescents with suicidal and non-suicidal self-harm, especially in the prevalence, methods, frequency and severity of suicidal thinking and depression, although the quality of the studies available precludes definitive conclusions.

Laboratory studies

There have been several reported studies of neurobiological indicators in people presenting with self-harm. These will be thoroughly reviewed in Chapter 4 in this book. However, at least partly due to the definitional differences, the results are hard to interpret and appear to be conflicting.

Crowell et al.[75] investigated measures of physiological reactivity in a sample of parasuicidal adolescent females (n = 23) who reported self-harm with suicidal, non-suicidal and ambivalent intent. These authors found reduced respiratory sinus arrhythmia (RSA) at baseline, greater RSA reactivity during negative mood induction, and attenuated peripheral serotonin levels compared with control subjects.

In a study of young women with borderline personality disorder (BPD) (n = 21) Ebner-Priemer et al.[76] showed that the BPD group had a significantly higher startle response than the control subjects in the electromyogram (showing amygdalar hyperarousal). Again the participants were not exclusively non-suicidal self-harmers. A more specific study by Nock and Mendes[72] investigated measures of physiological arousal in a group of adolescents presenting with non-suicidal self-injury (NSSI) (n = 62), showing higher physiological reactivity (skin conductance) during a distressing task. The results are interesting in that the higher physiological reactivity has not been shown in Crowell et al.'s study, raising a possibility that subjects with non-suicidal self-harm differ in this respect from others. It is not clear, however, from the study description if the authors specifically excluded those with suicidal self-harm.

Very few studies did head-to-head comparisons of the subjects with suicidal and non-suicidal self-harm. Where this was done, similar underlying neurobiological mechanisms were implicated.[77]

In summary, there is not enough evidence to draw a firm line between these two categories on the basis of the laboratory experiments; however, this area of study is relatively new and it may be that more evidence of neurobiological differences will be found.

Specific exclusion criteria

There are no specific exclusion criteria between suicidal and non-suicidal self-harmers beyond the definitions themselves (i.e. non-suicidal individuals would be excluded from a definition of suicidal self-harm and vice versa).

Follow-up studies

There are no direct follow-up comparison studies of suicidal and non-suicidal self-harmers, although both appear to be at elevated risk of suicide.[28] Most follow-up studies currently available do not directly distinguish between suicidal versus non-suicidal self-harmers[10,28,60,78] and thus an increased risk of completed suicide is yet to be demonstrated in purely non-suicidal self-harm samples. Both groups, however, are at a higher risk of subsequent suicide attempts.[37,78]

The prediction of further self-harm episodes and suicidal thinking has traditionally been achieved by means of a clinical assessment. A new paradigm proposed by Nock and Banaji[79] was devised to provide a laboratory-based test for predicting future suicide attempts by measuring a subject's implicit associations with self-injury.

Interestingly, although both authors support differentiation between suicidal and non-suicidal self-harm, the stimulus used to measure implicit associations was cutting – traditionally associated with non-suicidal self-injury. The test did, incidentally, accurately predict suicidal ideation at 6 months' follow-up.

Genetic/family studies

There are numerous studies supporting a genetic basis for self-harm. These will be reviewed in Chapter 3 of this book. Most of the studies relate to suicidal samples and the genetics of non-suicidal self-harm appears to be entirely virgin territory. There are no direct comparisons between suicidal versus non-suicidal self-harming individuals at present.

Deliberate self-injury syndrome

On the basis of the differences between some aspects of suicidal and non-suicidal behaviour a new category of deliberate self-injury syndrome (DSIS) has been proposed[57] based on previous research and definitions.[1,55,57] Central features of the syndrome include non-suicidal intent and feelings of tension, accompanied by a strong urge to hurt oneself and a sense of relief after self-harm. There must have been at least five episodes of self-harm causing significant distress or impairment. Exclusion criteria include psychosis, transsexualism, mental retardation, developmental disorders or a general medical condition. More research is required to characterise this syndrome further. The proponents equally hope that creating a separate diagnostic category in the *Diagnostic and Statistical Manual* (DSM) will stimulate research into the condition.

Bridging the gap

What should be made of the discussion above? It would seem absurd to treat two near-lethal overdoses differently on the basis of the reported differences in intent. On the other hand, it would be equally absurd to treat a near-lethal hanging in the same way as a superficial scratch.

Perhaps the best theoretical framework described in recent years that sheds some light on this debate was proposed by Thomas Joiner.[80] In an attempt to identify those at greatest risk of suicide he describes three main domains: the feeling of being a burden on loved ones; the sense of isolation; and the learned ability to hurt oneself. The third of these factors is central and of most pertinence to the current debate. Joiner proposes that individuals who engage in non-suicidal or suicidal self-harm gradually lose their fear of death through the process of habituation. The fear of death is seen as a central factor preventing suicide in a human being. Although this theory cannot explain all suicides, it provides an exciting opportunity to create a bridge between the understanding of suicidal and non-suicidal behaviour.

Conclusion

On the basis of the discussion above, it is concluded that at present there is only limited evidence for different types of self-harm representing different diagnostic entities. Self-harm can be seen as a broad spectrum of behaviours and in this book the authors adopt the NICE definition of self-harm[51] as self-poisoning or self-injury, irrespective of the apparent purpose of the act (based on the Kreitman–Hawton–De Leo tradition), thus covering a broad spectrum of behaviours. Within this spectrum there is emerging evidence of more or less well-defined categories, NSSI being one of these. NSSI will be discussed separately in this book wherever such a separation appears evidence based.

References

1. Favazza AR. The coming of age of self-mutilation. *J Nerv Ment Dis* 1998;186(5):259–68.
2. Favazza AR, Favazza B. *Bodies under siege: self-mutilation in culture and psychiatry*. Baltimore, MD: Johns Hopkins University Press; 1987.

3. *The Holy Bible. 21st Century King James Version:* containing the Old Testament and the New Testament. Gary, SD: 21st Century King James Bible Publishers; 1994.

4. Menninger KA. *Man against himself.* Oxford, UK: Harcourt, Brace; 1938.

5. Stengel E. *Suicide and attempted suicide.* Oxford, UK: Penguin Books; 1964.

6. Canetto SS. Women and suicidal behavior: a cultural analysis. *Am J Orthopsychiatry* 2008;78(2):259–66.

7. Canetto SS, Lester D. *Women and suicidal behavior.* New York, NY: Springer Publishing Co; 1995.

8. Kreitman N, Philip AE, Greer S, Bagley CR. Parasuicide. *Br J Psychiatry* 1969;115:746–7.

9. Hjelmeland H, Hawton K, Nordvik H, *et al.* Why people engage in parasuicide: a cross-cultural study of intentions. *Suicide Life Threat Behav* 2002;32:380–93.

10. Hjelmeland H, Stiles TC, Bille-Brahe U, *et al.* Parasuicide: the value of suicidal intent and various motives as predictors of future suicidal behaviour. *Arch Suicide Res* 1998;4(3):209–25.

11. Schmidtke A, Bille-Brahe U, DeLeo D, *et al.* Attempted suicide in Europe: rates, trends and sociodemographic characteristics of suicide attempters during the period 1989–1992. Results of the WHO/EURO Multicentre Study on Parasuicide. *Acta Psychiatr Scand* 1996 May;93:327–38.

12. Kehrer CA, Linehan MM. Interpersonal and emotional problem solving skills and parasuicide among women with borderline personality disorder. *J Pers Disord* 1996;10(2):153–63.

13. Beck A, Beck R, Kovacs M. Classification of suicidal behaviors: I. quantifying intent and medical lethality. *Am J Psychiatry* 1975;132:285–7.

14. Beck AT, Resnik HL, Lettieri DJ, editors. The prediction of suicide. Oxford, UK: Charles Press Publishers; 1974.

15. Silverman MM. The language of suicidology. *Suicide Life Threat Behav* 2006;36:519–32.

16. Hawton K, Harriss L, Hall S, *et al.* Deliberate self-harm in Oxford, 1990–2000: a time of change in patient characteristics. *Psychol Med* 2003;33(6):987–95.

17. Nock MK, Kessler RC. Prevalence of and risk factors for suicide attempts versus suicide gestures: analysis of the National Comorbidity Survey. *J Abnorm Psychol* 2006 Aug;115(3):616–23.

18. *Merriam-Webster Dictionary* [accessed 20 December 2008] Available from: http://www.merriam-webster.com.

19. Silverman MM, Berman AL, Sanddal ND, *et al.* Rebuilding the tower of Babel: a revised nomenclature for the study of suicide and suicidal behaviors. Part 2: suicide-related ideations, communications, and behaviors. *Suicide Life Threat Behav* 2007;37(3): 264–77.

20. Hjelmeland H, Knizek BL. Conceptual confusion about intentions and motives of nonfatal suicidal behavior: a discussion of terms employed in the literature of suicidology. *Arch Suicide Res* 1999;5(4):275–81.

21. Andriessen K. On 'intention' in the definition of suicide. *Suicide Life Threat Behav* 2006;36(5):533–8.

22. O'Carroll PW, Berman AL, Maris RW, *et al.* Beyond the Tower of Babel: a nomenclature for suicidology. *Suicide Life Threat Behav* 1996;26(3):237–52.

23. Posner K, Oquendo MA, Gould M, Stanley B, Davies M. Columbia Classification algorithm of suicide assessment (C-CASA): classification of suicidal events in the FDA's pediatric suicidal risk analysis of antidepressants. *Am J Psychiatry* 2007;164(7):1035–43.

24. Rudd MD. Suicidality in clinical practice: anxieties and answers. *J Clin Psychol* 2006;**62**(2):157–9.
25. Brent DA, Perper JA, Goldstein CE, *et al.* Risk factors for adolescent suicide. A comparison of adolescent suicide victims with suicidal inpatients. *Arch Gen Psychiatry* 1988;**45**(6):581–8.
26. Hawton K, van Heeringen K, editors. *The international handbook of suicide and attempted suicide.* New York, NY: John Wiley & Sons Ltd; 2000.
27. Brown GK, Henriques GR, Sosdjan D, Beck AT. Suicide intent and accurate expectations of lethality: predictors of medical lethality of suicide attempts. *J Consult Clin Psychol* 2004;**72**(6):1170–4.
28. Harriss L, Hawton K, Zahl D. Value of measuring suicidal intent in the assessment of people attending hospital following self-poisoning or self-injury. *Br J Psychiatry* 2005;**186**(1):60–6.
29. Guertin T, Lloyd-Richardson E, Spirito A, *et al.* Self-mutilative behavior in adolescents who attempt suicide by overdose. *J Am Acad Child Adolesc Psychiatry* 2001;**40**(9):1062–9.
30. Beck AT, Steer RA. Clinical predictors of eventual suicide: A 5- to 10-year prospective study of suicide attempters. *J Affect Disord* 1989;**17**(3):203–9.
31. Brown GK, Steer RA, Henriques GR, Beck AT. The internal struggle between the wish to die and the wish to live: a risk factor for suicide. *Am J Psychiatry* 2005;**162**(10):1977–9.
32. Kovacs M, Beck AT. The wish to die and the wish to live in attempted suicides. *J Clin Psychol* 1977;**33**(2):361–5.
33. Freeman DJ, Wilson K, Thigpen J, McGee RK. Assessing intention to die in self-injury behavior. In: Neuringer C, editor. *Psychological assessment of suicidal risk.* Oxford, UK: Charles C Thomas; 1974.
34. Meehan PJ, Lamb JA, Saltzman LE, O'Carroll PW. Attempted suicide among young adults: Progress toward a meaningful estimate of prevalence. *Am J Psychiatry* 1992;**149**(1):41–4.
35. Hawton K, Rodham K, Evans E, Weatherall R. Deliberate self harm in adolescents: self report survey in schools in England. *BMJ* 2002;**325**(7374):1207–11.
36. Walsh BW, Rosen PM. Self-mutilation: Theory, research, and treatment. New York, NY: Guilford Press; 1988.
37. Nock MK, Joiner TE, Jr, Gordon KH, Lloyd-Richardson E, Prinstein MJ. Non-suicidal self-injury among adolescents: diagnostic correlates and relation to suicide attempts. *Psychiatry Res* 2006;**144**(1):65–72.
38. Jacobs DG, editor. *The Harvard Medical School guide to suicide assessment and intervention.* San Francisco, CA: Jossey-Bass; 1999.
39. Maris RW, Berman AL, Maltsberger JT, Yufit RI. *Assessment and prediction of suicide.* New York, NY: Guilford Press; 1992.
40. Haw CM, Hawton K, Houston K, Townsend E. Correlates of relative lethality and suicidal intent among deliberate self-harm patients. *Suicide Life Threat Behav* 2003;**33**(4):353–64.
41. Douglas J, Cooper J, Amos T, *et al.* 'Near-fatal' deliberate self-harm: Characteristics, prevention and implications for the prevention of suicide. *J Affect Disord* 2004;**79**(1–3):263–8.
42. Skegg K. Self-harm. *Lancet* 2005;**366**(9495):1471–83.
43. Berman AL, Shepherd G, Silverman MM. The LSARS-II: Lethality of Suicide Attempt Rating Scale – updated. *Suicide Life Threat Behav* 2003;**33**(3):261–76.
44. Millstein SG, Halpern-Felsher BL. Perceptions of risk and vulnerability. *J Adolesc Health* 2002;**31**(Suppl 1):10–27.
45. Carter GL, Clover K, Whyte IM, *et al.* Postcards from the EDge project: randomised

controlled trial of an intervention using postcards to reduce repetition of hospital treated deliberate self poisoning. *BMJ* 2005;**331**(7520):805.

46. Harrington R, Kerfoot M, Dyer E, *et al.* Randomized trial of a home-based family intervention for children who have deliberately poisoned themselves. *J Am Acad Child Adolesc Psychiatry* 1998;**37**(5):512–8.

47. Hawton K, Harriss L, Simkin S, Bale E, Bond A. Self-cutting: patient characteristics compared with self-poisoners. *Suicide Life Threat Behav* 2004;**34**(3):199–208.

48. De Leo D, Burgis S, Bertolote JM, *et al.* Definitions of suicidal behavior: lessons learned from the WHO/EURO multicentre Study. *Crisis* 2006;**27**(1):4–15.

49. Brown GK, Jeglic E, Henriques GR, Beck AT. Cognitive therapy, cognition, and suicidal behavior. In: Ellis TE, editor. *Cognition and suicide: theory, research, and therapy.* Washington, DC: American Psychological Association; 2006: pp. 53–74.

50. Silverman MM, Berman AL, Sanddal ND, *et al.* Rebuilding the tower of Babel: a revised nomenclature for the study of suicide and suicidal behaviors. Part 1: background, rationale, and methodology. *Suicide Life Threat Behav* 2007;**37**(3):248–63.

51. National Collaborating Centre for Mental Health. *Self-harm: the short-term physical and psychological management and secondary prevention of self-harm in primary and secondary care.* Clinical Guideline 16. London: Gaskell and British Psychological Society; 2004.

52. De Leo D, Heller TS. Who are the kids who self-harm? An Australian self-report school survey. *Med J Aust* 2004;**181**(3):140–4.

53. Carter G, Reith DM, Whyte IM, McPherson M. Repeated self-poisoning: increasing severity of self-harm as a predictor of subsequent suicide. *Br J Psychiatry* 2005;**186**:253–7.

54. Feighner JP, Robins E, Guze SB, *et al.* Diagnostic criteria for use in psychiatric research. *Arch Gen Psychiatry* 1972;**26**(1):57–63.

55. Walsh BW. *Treating self-injury: a practical guide.* New York, NY: Guilford Press; 2006.

56. Pattison E, Kahan J. The deliberate self-harm syndrome. *Am J Psychiatry* 1983;**140**(7):867–72.

57. Muehlenkamp JJ. Self-injurious behavior as a separate clinical syndrome. *Am J Orthopsychiatry* 2005;**75**(2):324–33.

58. Hjelmeland H, Nordvik H, Bille-Brahe U, *et al.* A cross-cultural study of suicide intent in parasuicide patients. *Suicide Life Threat Behav* 2000;**30**(4):295–303.

59. Favazza AR, Conterio K. Female habitual self-mutilators. *Acta Psychiatr Scand* 1989;**79**(3):283–9.

60. Hawton K, Harriss L. Deliberate self-harm by under-15-year-olds: Characteristics, trends and outcome. *J Child Psychol Psychiatry* 2008;**49**(4):441–8.

61. Muehlenkamp JJ, Gutierrez PM. An investigation of differences between self-injurious behavior and suicide attempts in a sample of adolescents. *Suicide Life Threat Behav* 2004;**34**(1):12–23.

62. Muehlenkamp JJ, Gutierrez PM. Risk for suicide attempts among adolescents who engage in non-suicidal self-injury. *Arch Suicide Res* 2007;**11**(1):69–82.

63. Eaton DK, Kann L, Kinchen S, *et al.* Youth Risk Behavior Surveillance United States, 2007 [accessed 20 December 2008] Available from: http://www.cdc.gov/mmwr/preview/mmwrhtml/ss5704a1.htm.

64. Sarkar P, Sattar FA, Gode N, Basannar DR. Failed suicide and deliberate self-harm: A need for specific nomenclature. *Indian J Psychiatry* 2006;**48**:78–83

65. Gratz KL. Measurement of deliberate self-harm: preliminary data on the Deliberate Self-Harm Inventory. *J Psychopathol Behav Assess* 2001;**23**(4):253–63.

66. Ross S, Heath N. A study of the frequency of self-mutilation in a community sample of adolescents. *J Youth Adolesc* 2002;31(1):67–77.

67. Nock MK, Borges G, Bromet EJ, *et al.* Suicide and suicidal behavior. *Epidemiol Rev* 2008 July 24, 2008:mxn002.

68. Jacobson CM, Muehlenkamp JJ, Miller AL, Turner JB. Psychiatric impairment among adolescents engaging in different types of deliberate self-harm. *J Clin Child Adolesc Psychol* 2008;37(2):363–75.

69. Zoroglu SS, Tuzun U, Sar V, *et al.* Suicide attempt and self-mutilation among Turkish high school students in relation with abuse, neglect and dissociation. *Psychiatry Clin Neurosci* 2003;57(1):119–26.

70. Pollock LR, Williams J. Problem solving and suicidal behavior. *Suicide Life Threat Behav* 1998;28(4):375–87.

71. Pollock LR, Williams J. Effective problem solving in suicide attempters depends on specific autobiographical recall. *Suicide Life Threat Behav* 2001;31(4):386–96.

72. Nock MK, Mendes WB, Nock MK, Mendes WB. Physiological arousal, distress tolerance, and social problem-solving deficits among adolescent self-injurers. *J Consult Clin Psychol* 2008;76(1):28–38.

73. Najmi S, Wegner DM, Nock MK, *et al.* Thought suppression and self-injurious thoughts and behaviors. *Behav Res Ther* 2007;45(8):1957–65.

74. Nock MK, Wedig MM, Holmberg EB, Hooley JM. The emotion reactivity scale: development, evaluation, and relation to self-injurious thoughts and behaviors. *Behav Ther* 2008;39(2):107–16.

75. Crowell SE, Beauchaine TP, McCauley E, *et al.* Psychological, autonomic, and serotonergic correlates of parasuicide among adolescent girls. *Dev Psychopathol* 2005;17(4):1105–27.

76. Ebner-Priemer UW, Badeck S, Beckmann C, *et al.* Affective dysregulation and dissociative experience in female patients with borderline personality disorder: a startle response study. *J Psychiatr Res* 2005;39(1):85–92.

77. New AS, Trestman RL, Mitropoulou V, *et al.* Serotonergic function and self-injurious behavior in personality disorder patients. *Psychiatry Res* 1997;69(1):17–26.

78. Hawton K, Harriss L. Deliberate self-harm in young people: characteristics and subsequent mortality in a 20-year cohort of patients presenting to hospital. *J Clin Psychiatry* 2007;68(10):1574–83.

79. Nock MK, Banaji MR. Prediction of suicide ideation and attempts among adolescents using a brief performance-based test. *J Consult Clin Psychol* 2007;75(5):707–15.

80. Joiner T. *Why people die by suicide*. Cambridge, MA: Harvard University Press; 2005.

CHAPTER 2

PREVALENCE AND NATURAL HISTORY OF SELF-HARM

Dennis Ougrin
Marinos Kyriakopoulos

Introduction

How common is self-harm? The answer to this question is not straightforward. It depends on the definition of self-harm – whether researchers want to establish the prevalence of suicide attempts, suicidal and non-suicidal self-harm or just non-suicidal self-harm,[1] detection tools – whether these are anonymised, self-reported or interviewer-administered;[2] survey type – cross-sectional, retrospective or prospective;[1,3] informants – usually either adolescents or their parents,[1,3] age of participants[4] and population studied – general population, clinical population (inpatients or outpatients) or adolescents presenting to emergency departments.[3] Finally, prevalence will depend on the time frame covered, e.g. whether lifetime, last 12 months or current self-harm is enquired about.

The reported lifetime prevalence of self-harm varies significantly depending on the interplay of the factors above. The available published figures range between 4 per cent[5] in the general adult population and 82 per cent[6] in adolescent psychiatric inpatients.

The optimal approach to establishing the prevalence of self-harm should follow these steps. First, a clear definition of self-harm should be established. Second, the age of the adolescents and the time frame covered need to be specified. Third, a survey should be done on a representative sample of the adolescents in the general population using self-report, anonymised and validated questionnaires. This approach is probably best for addressing issues such as needs assessment, service planning and preventative interventions. Having said this, the methodology of the prevalence estimates may vary depending on the purpose of the survey. For instance, service commissioners might like to know the proportion of the total number of adolescents referred to child and adolescent mental health services who self-harm, or treating clinicians might be interested in the parental recognition of self-harm.

One of the most important factors in interpreting the results of a self-harm prevalence survey is the tool used. Using different tools in similar populations may result in reports of very different prevalence rates indeed (40.2 per cent using the Deliberate Self-harm Inventory (DSHI) versus 6.6 per cent using the Lifestyle and Coping Questionnaire (LaCQ).[7,8] The questions asked in surveys of self-harm prevalence vary from a single yes/no question to lengthy semi-structured interviews. In general, the larger the sample under investigation the simpler the tool used. Below is a brief review of the tools used for establishing the prevalence of self-harm. These tools are different from the tools used to measure risk, assess self-harm in-depth for clinical or research reasons, or measure changes in self-harm over time.[9-11] The overlap, however, between the uses of these tools is considerable: some screening tools might be used for clinical reasons and vice versa.

Examples of the tools currently available are discussed below.

Detection tools

The tools most commonly used to establish the prevalence of self-harm are self-report questionnaires or interviewer-administered schedules.

Structured and semi-structured interviews

The most commonly used structured and semi-structured interviews have items designed to identify suicidality. However, the wording of the questions varies significantly. Below is a comparison of the items designed to measure suicidality in some commonly used schedules (Table 2.1).

Most interviews have versions for young people and informants (parents). In Table 2.1 the authors focused on the young people-oriented versions of the instruments as these are more likely to produce accurate prevalence data. Since the time covered by the questions varies from instrument to instrument, this was not included in the table. Most instruments, however, cover the entire lifetime and the previous year, with the previous 6 months, previous month and 'recent' self-harm being assessed more rarely.[19]

It is plain from Table 2.1 that different tools are likely to yield different prevalence rates for self-harm and wider suicidality. The main differences are in the breadth of behaviours, the wording used and the thresholds for identifying the presence of the behaviour. The childhood and adolescent psychiatric assessment (CAPA) interview glossary, for instance, provides specific definitions for a broad range of behaviours and thoughts. Suicidal thoughts are defined as 'thinking specifically about killing oneself, by whatever means', suicide attempts as 'episodes of deliberate self-harmful behaviour, or potentially self-harmful behaviour, involving some intention to die at the time of the attempt'; non-suicidal self-damaging acts as 'self-mutilation or other potentially self-damaging acts (e.g. wrist-slashing, cigarette burns) not accompanied by any wish or intention to die'; and finally 'suicidal' behaviour without intent defined as 'actions threatening suicide, without intention of ending life'. There are also specific definitions

Table 2.1 Questions enquiring about suicidality in selected interviewer-administered schedules

Tool	Suicidal self-harm	Non-suicidal self-harm	Any self-harm	Thoughts about suicide or self-harm
K-SADS-PL	Have you actually tried to kill yourself?		Did you ever try to hurt yourself?	Sometimes children who get upset or feel bad think about dying or even killing themselves. Have you ever had such thought?
DAWBA			Did you try to harm yourself or kill yourself?	Did you think about harming yourself or killing yourself?
DISC	Have you ever, in your whole life, tried to kill yourself or made a suicide attempt?		[In the last year] was there a time when you thought seriously about killing yourself?	
CAPA	Have you actually tried to kill yourself? Have you done anything that made other people think you wanted to die?	Have you ever hurt yourself on purpose (apart from when you wanted to die?) or cut yourself on purpose?		Have you thought about actually killing yourself?
DICA	Did you try to kill yourself?			Have you thought about killing yourself?
ESRAIDA			Have you ever hurt yourself or tried to kill yourself?	Have you ever seriously thought about killing yourself? By seriously, I mean every day for a week, or more?

CAPA, Child and Adolescent Psychiatric Assessment;[17] DAWBA, Development and Wellbeing Assessment;[13,14] DICA, Diagnostic Interview for Children and Adolescents;[16] DISC, Diagnostic Interview Schedule for Children;[15] ESRAIDA, Evaluation of Suicide Risk Among Adolescents and Imminent Danger Assessment;[18] K-SADS-PL, The Kiddie-Schedule for Affective Disorders and Schizophrenia Present and Lifetime Version.[12]
The authors would like to thank the copyright holders of the relevant instruments for their kind permission to reproduce these questions: Dr A. Angold, Dr P. Fisher, Dr J. Kaufman, Dr R. Goodman, Dr W. Reich and Dr M. Rotheram-Borus.

for thinking about death, suicidal plans, suicidal intent and the factors associated with self-harm. In contrast, the DISC questions are specifically focused on suicidal thoughts and behaviours. Interviews also differ on the thresholds used for coding self-harm. K-SADS-PL, for example, has a very high threshold for identification of both self-harm and suicidal thinking. In order to qualify for a threshold coding the young person must report thinking of suicide often and having thought of a specific method. The coding threshold for suicide attempts requires definite suicidal intent, and the threshold for non-suicidal self-harm requires either a frequency of more than four in a year or serious injury, like scarring. The epidemiological version of this tool (K-SADS-E) has less specific questions designed to increase sensitivity. In contrast in the DAWBA, 'yes' answers to broadly formulated questions on suicidal thoughts and behaviour are sufficient for a clinical coding. The tools that only enquire about suicidal self-harm are likely to miss out on a large proportion of the young people with non-suicidal self-harm. Finally, the inclusion of the word 'serious' in the questions may lead to underestimation of self-harm.

Self-report questionnaires

Some of the commonly used self-report questionnaires and their relevant items are presented in Table 2.2. These are frequently used in prevalence estimations of suicidality.

Many questionnaires used for screening 'suicidality' do not in fact have items measuring self-harm behaviours and suicidal ideation is used as a proxy measure. The questionnaires that do measure self-harm mostly screen for suicide attempts, and there are very few measures that adequately screen for suicidal and non-suicidal self-harm. This is perhaps the reason why many researchers use brief, non-validated tools in their studies, e.g. 'Have you harmed or hurt your body on purpose (for example, cutting or burning your skin, hitting yourself, or pulling out your hair)?'[4] or an option of 'Hurt myself on purpose' in response to the question 'How do you deal with stress?'[28] Both suicidal and non-suicidal self-harm are likely to be reported in response to these questions.

Alternatively, some authors use tools designed primarily for the functional assessment of self-harm, in order to ascertain self-harm prevalence, e.g. the Functional Assessment of Self-Mutilation (FASM).[29,30] Using FASM seems to be associated with consistently higher estimates of the prevalence of self-harm, perhaps because of the breadth of the behaviours covered (including tattooing and picking on the wound). Yet some of the typical self-harm behaviours, like overdosing, are not included, presumably because of their association with suicidal self-harm. FASM allows for the differentiation between suicidal and non-suicidal self-harm. Similar problems might arise with the use of the Deliberate Self-harm Inventory (DSHI).[8]

The Self-harm Behaviour Questionnaire[31] has recently been studied in adolescent samples.[32] It allows the study of both suicidal and non-suicidal self-harm. Further evidence is required for its use in clinical populations.

Table 2.2 Questions enquiring about suicidality in selected self-report questionnaires

Tool	Thoughts about suicide or self-harm	Suicidal self-harm	Non-suicidal self-harm	Any self-harm
YSR	I think about killing myself			I deliberately try to hurt or kill myself
MFQ	I thought about killing myself			
YRBS	Did you ever seriously consider attempting suicide? Did you make a plan about how you would attempt suicide?	How many times did you actually attempt suicide?		
LaCQ	Have you during the past month or the past year seriously thought about taking an overdose or trying to harm yourself but not actually done so?			Have you ever deliberately taken an overdose (e.g. of pills or other medication) or tried to harm yourself in some other way (such as cut yourself)?
SBQ	Have you ever thought about or attempted to kill yourself?			
HASS	[How often] have you had ideas about killing yourself?	[How often] have you tried to kill yourself?		
DSHI			Have you ever intentionally (i.e., on purpose) cut your wrist, arms, or other area(s) of your body (without intending to kill yourself)?*	

*The question is repeated with 16 other behaviours in the original version and with 9 behaviours in a short version (DSHI-9).

DSH, Deliberate Self-harm Inventory;[8,27] HASS, Harkavy Asnis Suicide Scale;[26] LaCQ, Lifestyle and Coping Questionnaire;[24] MFQ, Mood and Feelings Questionnaire;[20] SBQ, Suicide Behavior Questionnaire;[25] YRBS, Youth Risk Behavior Survey;[23] YSR, Youth Self Report.[21,22]

The authors would like to thank the copyright holders of the relevant instruments for their kind permission to reproduce these questions: Dr T. Achenbach, Dr A. Angold, Dr K. Gratz, Dr J. Harkavy-Friedman, Dr K. Hawton and Dr M. Linehan.

The Lifestyle and Coping Questionnaire[24] was used in the largest prevalence study of self-harm to date. It also allows for the differentiation between suicidal and non-suicidal self-harm. The full questionnaire has 97 items and its psychometric properties have not yet been reported.

Prevalence of self-harm

The most comprehensive review of the prevalence of self-harm to date[3] included 128 studies comprising 513,188 adolescents. A particular value of this review lies in it being an attempt to collate prevalence data for different kinds of self-harm, including attempted suicide with clear intent to die and self-injury with or without such intent. The authors of the review also did not limit their search to the English language, broadening the population base significantly. The mean proportion of adolescents reporting lifetime prevalence of attempted suicide across the studies was 9.7 per cent (95% CI 8.5–10.9) with 6.4 per cent (95% CI 5.4–7.5) reporting a suicide attempt in the previous year, and 29.9 per cent (95% CI 26.1–33.8) reporting lifetime suicidal thoughts; 13.2 per cent (95% CI 8.1–18.3) reported engaging in deliberate self-harm at some point in their lifetime, although some of the estimates were as high as 26 per cent within the previous year. Big differences among the studies probably arise primarily from the studies' methodology and the population studied. There was also significant within-group variation beyond that expected by chance, again pointing to significant differences in the methodology and/or populations. A consistent finding across several studies was a greater prevalence of suicide attempts in North America versus Europe (lifetime prevalence 12.9 per cent vs 6.9 per cent, respectively, $p = 0.001$). A somewhat surprising finding was a lower prevalence of suicidal phenomena in Asian adolescents, consistent with recent reports of a lower suicide rate in young Asian males, but not females.[33]

The relationship between ethnicity and self-harm is by no means straightforward. It is possible that suicidal phenomena in ethnic minorities are higher in areas where minority groups are smaller[34] and where traditional lifestyles have been eroded.

Since the publication of the review, several more studies attempting to establish self-harm prevalence have been undertaken. The most notable of these is the Child & Adolescent Self-Harm in Europe (CASE) study.[24] Over 30,000 mainly 15- and 16-year-olds were studied in Australia, Belgium, Hungary, Ireland, the Netherlands, Norway and the UK, using the LaCQ. Overall, 13.5 per cent of females and 4.3 per cent of males reported an episode of self-harm meeting the strict study criteria (based on Hawton's definition, please see chapter 1 for in-depth discussion) in their lifetime and 8.9 per cent of females and 2.6 per cent of males reported an episode meeting the study criteria in the past year. Significant variations in the lifetime prevalence of strictly defined adolescent self-harm were reported across six different countries in Europe and Australia (male rates ranging between 2.4 per cent in the Netherlands and 6.5 per cent in Belgium, female rates between 5.7 per cent in the Netherlands and 17 per cent in Australia). The study examined the reported intent of self-harm in detail. Overall, 59 per cent of the subjects reported a wish to die as either a sole or one of the reasons for the self-harm. Intent to die was reported as the only reason by 3.9 per cent of the adolescents, again demonstrating difficulties with clear differentiation between the suicidal and non-suicidal groups. On the other hand, there was a large purely non-suicidal group in this study. The authors did not present comparative characteristics of suicidal and non-suicidal groups, but this may form the basis of further publications. An advantage of this study is the use of standardised assessment tools, studying similar populations under similar conditions and a big sample size. One important disadvantage is that the results cannot be compared with similar studies from other researchers using other detection tools or using different definitions of self-harm.

There have also been recent reports of epidemiological studies of self-harm from Japan[35] (lifetime prevalence 9.9 per cent, $n = 2974$, m < f, using a non-validated single question design) and Canada[36] (lifetime prevalence 16.9 per cent $n = 568$, m < f, using a modified version of the LaCQ). The definition used was narrower and suicidal acts were specifically excluded. A study in Finland[37] found the lifetime prevalence of self-cutting to be 11.5 per cent and of other self-harm 10.2 per cent, ($n = 4205$, aged 13–18 years f > m, using a non-validated single-question questionnaire).

In the USA, an excellent source of data on the prevalence of self-harm is The Youth Risk Behavior Surveillance System (YRBSS). A 53-item survey that monitors six categories of health-risk behaviours is administered to large representative populations of high-school students. These surveys have been conducted since 1991. The survey is focused primarily on self-reported behaviours that are likely to result in unintentional injuries and violence, tobacco use, alcohol and other drug use, sexual behaviours likely to contribute to unintended pregnancy and sexually transmitted diseases, unhealthy diet and physical inactivity. In addition, the YRBSS monitors the prevalence of obesity and asthma.

The latest data from the Youth Risk Behavior Survey (2008) ($n = 14,103$) indicated that in the previous 12 months 14.5 per cent (m < f) of students had seriously considered attempting suicide, 11.3 per cent (m < f) had made a suicidal plan, 6.9 per cent of young people attempted suicide (m < f) and of those 2 per cent sought medical or nursing care (m < f). Although the wording of the question in the YRBS enquiring about self-harm ('During the past 12 months, how many times did you actually attempt suicide?') is designed to only include suicidal self-harm, further studies of this group revealed a large subset of individuals with non-suicidal intent.[38]

Self-harm in specific populations

Self-harm is very prevalent in psychiatric outpatients and especially inpatients.[39] It is also very common in socially disadvantaged and marginalised populations. For instance up to 57.5 per cent of homeless adolescents had a history of self-harm and 25 per cent reported at least one suicide attempt in an Austrian study where $n = 40$, age 14–23 years, using the Structured Clinical Interview for DSM (SCID).[40] In a Scottish sample ($n = 1258$, age 19 years, using the DISC) strong identification with Goth subculture conferred a risk of lifetime self-harm and attempted suicide of 53 per cent and 47 per cent, respectively;[41] homo- and bisexual individuals appeared to be at least twice as likely to have attempted suicide than the general population.[42] Self-harm is also very prevalent among incarcerated youths, with 12.4 per cent reporting a prior suicide attempt, 30 per cent suicidal ideation and/or behaviour and 30 per cent reporting self-harm behaviours while incarcerated.[43]

Non-suicidal self-injury

Prevalence studies of non-suicidal self-injury in adolescents are relatively new, with most large studies undertaken only in the past 10 years.

Those authors who study adolescent non-suicidal self-injury (NSSI) separately from suicide attempts report large variability in the lifetime prevalence in recent studies: 7.5 per cent,[4] $n = 508$, age 10–14 years, m = f, using a self-report non-validated questionnaire; 13.9 per cent,[28] $n = 440$, average age 14 years, m < f, using a non-validated screening questionnaire followed by a semi-structured interview; 15 per cent,[44] $n = 424$, mean age 15.3 years, m < f, using a self-report non-validated questionnaire; 15.9 per cent,[45] $n = 390$, mean age 16.3 years, m < f, using an unpublished Self-harmful Behavior Scale (also 5.9 per cent reported attempted suicide independent of non-suicidal self-injury); 21.4 per cent[46] $n = 862$, age 14–17 years, m = f, using a non-validated self-report questionnaire (lifetime prevalence of suicidal attempts was 10.1 per cent, m < f); 37.2 per cent[30] using FASM, ninth to twelfth grade, m < f; 40.2 per cent,[8] $n = 140$, age 14 years, m < f (but not statistically significant) using the DSHI-9; 46.5 per cent,[29] $n = 633$, average age 15.5 years, m = f, using the FASM (7 per cent reported a history of suicide attempt).

It is not entirely clear why the studies report these significantly different rates, but the age of the population studied and the tool used (especially the range of self-harm behaviours enquired about) are perhaps the most important sources of difference.

Another observation of interest is that older studies seem to report consistently lower prevalence of NSSI. For example, a study conducted in 1993[47] reported a 2.5 per cent prevalence of NSSI during the previous year and a 1997 study 5.1 per cent.[48] Whether this reflects a true increase in prevalence, or methodological differences are responsible, is unclear.

Recent studies indicate that non-suicidal self-harm is prevalent in high-functioning individuals, for example students of American elite universities[49] and young people from high socioeconomic classes,[30] the groups not traditionally associated with self-harm. These findings, coupled with the high prevalence rates reported by the studies, led some authors to call self-harm a spreading epidemic.[50]

Hospital presentations

Hospital presentations with self-harm have been studied extensively, although it is clear that the adolescents who present with self-harm to emergency departments are different from those who self-harm in the community in important ways, especially the method of self-harm (primarily overdose in hospital presentations versus self-injury in community samples).

One of the most comprehensive systems of self-harm registration is that administered by the National Center for Injury Prevention and Control in Atlanta, Georgia, part of the Centers for Disease Control and Prevention (CDC) in the USA. Interestingly, the definition used by the CDC does not differentiate between suicidal and non-suicidal self-harm. Self-harm is defined as 'Injury or poisoning resulting from a deliberate violent act inflicted on oneself with the intent to take one's own life or with the intent to harm oneself. This category includes suicide, suicide attempt, and other intentional self-injuries.'[51]

Reports on self-harm presentations to emergency departments throughout the USA are available on the National Center for Injury Prevention and Control website via the Web-based Injury Statistics Query and Reporting System (WISQARS).[52] The number of adolescents presenting to emergency departments with intentional self-injuries appears to have increased in the USA. For example, the rate of self-harm (per 100,000 population) in 10- to 14-year-olds has increased from 76 in 2001 to 99 in 2007. The increase was especially striking in girls (119 vs 157, respectively). In 15- to 19-year-olds self-harm increased less dramatically, from 301/100,000 in 2001 to 323/100,000 in 2007. Again the increase was much greater among girls (392/100,000 in 2001, 435/100,000 in 2007).

In Britain, a similar system exists in Oxford, administered by the Centre for Suicide Research. It allows for a much finer characterisation of the patients presenting with self-harm but lacks the power and representativeness of the CDC. There was some evidence of the numbers reaching a plateau in the past 3 years, but overall a strikingly similar trend towards increased adolescent self-harm presentations was reported for the period of 2000–6,[53] again with an overall increase especially prominent amongst teenage girls.

What is the natural history and outcome of self-harm?

The onset of self-harm has traditionally been associated with the early teens, on average around the age of 13 years,[6] peaking in the late teens and gradually reducing in adulthood. Cross-sectional studies seem to confirm this pattern;[53] however, recent studies indicate that self-harm may already be prevalent in pre-adolescents.[4] The risk of self-harm repetition is in the region of 5–15 per cent per year,[54] although the risk of repetition of non-suicidal self-harm may be much greater.

Hospital presentation with self-harm is associated with an increased risk of death from all causes and especially suicide.[55,56] After a mean follow-up period of just over 11 years, 1.1 per cent of under-15-year-olds had died by probable suicide.[56] In 15- to 19-year-olds this figure was around 1.5 per cent.[55] Males are more likely to complete suicide and most suicides occur soon after the index hospital presentation with self-harm.

Few large long-term longitudinal cohorts exist to answer the question about how self-harm changes over time. One exception to this is a large (n = 1265) birth cohort in New Zealand followed up for 25 years.[57] The participants were asked (using a non-validated questionnaire) to report suicidal thoughts and behaviour. Those adolescents who reported suicidal thoughts or behaviour were much more likely to have suicidal thoughts and behaviour in young adulthood as well as major depression. An association with a range of psychiatric disorders in adulthood was demonstrated in a sample of 593 subjects followed up for 7 years.[58] A 6-year follow-up study of 132 adolescents who deliberately poisoned themselves between the ages of 11 and 16 years found 39 (30 per cent) harmed themselves deliberately at least once after leaving school, although self-harm ceased in most cases within 3 years. Those who continued to self-harm had greater psychopathology and were exposed to a greater number of adverse events. Longitudinal studies of non-suicidal self-harm in adolescents are absent.[59]

Is the prevalence of self-harm rising?

Self-harm as measured by the Youth Risk Behavior Survey in the USA (the specific question regarding self-harm in the survey is 'During the past 12 months, how many times did you actually attempt suicide?') appears to indicate a decrease in the prevalence of attempted suicide in the past 26 years.[60,61]

During 1991–2007, a significant decrease occurred in the percentage of young people who seriously considered attempting suicide (29.0 per cent to 14.5 per cent) and in the percentage of students who made a suicide plan (18.6 per cent to 11.3 per cent), although interestingly the proportion of the ideators who also make plans seems to have increased. The percentage of young people who attempted suicide, however, did not change significantly during 1991–2007 (7.3 per cent to 6.9 per cent). This finding is of interest as it did not seem to mirror a significant reduction in suicides over the same period. The percentage of students who made a suicide attempt that required medical attention increased slightly during 1991–2007 (1.7 per cent to 2 per cent). During 2005–7, significant decreases occurred in the percentage of students who seriously considered attempting suicide (16.9 per cent to 14.5 per cent), made a suicide plan (13.0 per cent to 11.3 per cent) and who attempted suicide (8.4 per cent to 6.9 per cent).

A common method of trying to capture secular trends is to study the same population using the same assessment methods at different time points. Using anonymous self-report measures would appear to be the ideal way of measuring secular changes in adolescent self-harm. There are few studies employing this methodology. A Dutch study[62] (1993, $n = 2719$, age 4–18 years; 2003, $n = 2567$ age 6–18 years, using a single question requiring a yes/no answer including suicidal and non-suicidal self-harm) found an increase in lifetime self-harm in girls only (boys 1.7 per cent vs 1.3 per cent, girls 3.1 per cent vs 6.5 per cent). American community-based studies indicate that the prevalence of self-harm is likely to be rising. Repeat surveys of similar populations are rare and where available tend to indicate an increase.[32,45,63,64]

Completed suicide

No discussion of prevalence would be complete without a discussion of completed suicide. The link between self-harm and suicide is well established, although the link between non-suicidal self-harm and suicide remains to be shown.

The World Health Organization (WHO) reports on suicide rates across the globe. The most recent statistics on youth suicide,[65] as summarised by the WHO in two age groups (5–14 years and 15–24 years), are presented in Table 2.3, with the year of the most recent data for each country also noted.

Suicide rates seem to be particularly high in the Russian Federation and other former Soviet states, Finland and New Zealand and relatively low in Mediterranean countries, Kuwait and the UK. In most countries, young males are more likely to commit suicide than females (Table 2.3). This may be due to males being associated with more risk factors, including a higher lethality of the method employed.[64,65] Interestingly, more female than male adolescent and young adult suicides have been recorded in the mainland and selected urban and rural areas of China (Table 2.3); the large number of suicides in young Chinese rural women seem to account for this finding.[68] In addition, late adolescent suicides are much more prevalent than early adolescent and child suicides, which has been related to the increasing prevalence of depressive disorders and substance misuse in adolescence. A history of previous suicide attempt is the most significant risk factor for completed suicide, increasing the risk 30 times in males and three times in females.[65] In a recent UK study[69] suicide rates in 10- to 19-year-old youths over a 7-year period (1997–2003) correspond to an average rate of 3.28 per 100,000 per year, with marked gender differences (males:females = 4.79:1.69) in this age group. There is evidence of a 30 per cent decline in male but not female suicides during the study period while the overall suicide rate for 15- to 19-year-olds was more than 12 times higher than that for 10- to 14-year-olds.

Table 2.3 Youth suicide rates per 100,000 population in selected countries by gender and age (from the World Health Organization website, 2008)

Country	5–14 years			15–24 years			Year
	Male	Female	All	Male	Female	All	
Australia	0.5	0.5	0.5	17.4	3.6	10.7	2003
Austria	0.2	0.0	0.1	14.8	3.2	9.1	2006
Belarus	1.8	0.5	1.2	34.6	5.8	20.5	2003
Brazil	0.3	0.3	0.3	6.9	2.4	4.6	2002
Bulgaria	1.3	0.8	1.1	7.3	2.3	4.9	2004
Canada	0.8	0.6	0.7	17.0	4.8	11.0	2004
China	0.9	0.8	0.8	5.4	8.6	6.9	1999
Hong Kong	0.3	0.0	0.1	11.4	7.2	9.3	2005
Croatia	0.8	0.0	0.4	13.1	3.1	8.2	2005
Czech Republic	0.7	0.4	0.6	12.2	2.4	7.4	2005
Estonia	1.4	0.0	0.7	25.2	4.9	15.2	2005
Finland	1.0	0.3	0.6	32.2	5.9	19.4	2006
France	0.6	0.2	0.4	11.0	3.3	7.2	2005
Germany	0.4	0.2	0.3	10.5	2.7	6.7	2004
Greece	0.0	0.2	0.1	3.1	0.6	1.9	2006
Hungary	0.9	0.0	0.5	12.0	2.6	7.4	2005
Ireland	0.7	0.4	0.5	20.4	3.2	11.9	2005
Israel	0.5	0.0	0.2	10.9	0.9	6.0	2003
Italy	0.2	0.1	0.2	6.2	1.3	3.8	2003
Japan	0.9	0.3	0.7	18.2	9.7	14.1	2006
Kuwait	0.0	0.0	0.0	1.2	0.0	0.6	2002
Latvia	3.3	0.9	2.1	24.5	3.4	14.2	2005
Lithuania	0.9	0.5	0.7	37.1	4.2	21.0	2005
Luxemburg	0.0	0.0	0.0	22.1	0.0	11.3	2005
Mexico	0.9	0.5	0.7	10.3	2.8	6.4	2005
Netherlands	0.7	0.2	0.5	7.3	2.6	5.0	2004
Norway	1.3	0.3	0.8	17.2	7.2	12.3	2005
New Zealand	1.0	0.3	0.7	30.4	5.7	18.2	2000
Poland	1.1	0.3	0.7	19.8	2.3	11.2	2005
Portugal	0.0	0.0	0.0	5.6	1.6	3.7	2003
Russian Federation	2.8	1.0	1.9	46.5	7.5	27.3	2005
Serbia	0.5	0.0	0.3	10.6	3.0	6.9	2006
Slovakia	0.0	0.3	0.2	13.0	1.7	7.5	2005
Slovenia	0.0	0.0	0.0	15.7	5.6	10.8	2006
Spain	0.2	0.2	0.2	6.1	1.5	3.9	2005
Sweden	0.7	0.5	0.6	14.6	4.5	9.7	2002
Switzerland	0.5	0.0	0.2	15.4	5.3	10.5	2005
Ukraine	2.0	0.3	1.1	22.8	3.8	13.5	2005
United Kingdom	0.1	0.1	0.1	7.4	2.3	4.9	2005
USA	1.0	0.3	0.7	16.1	3.5	10.0	2005

Summary

In summary, self-harm in adolescence is common and associated with a variety of negative psychosocial outcomes in adulthood. The majority of adolescents who self-harm will not self-harm in adulthood. However, a large minority will continue to self-harm and a small minority will commit suicide. Detection of the true prevalence of self-harm is fraught with definitional and methodological difficulties. There is a puzzling picture of trends in self-harm in recent years. On one hand there has been a consistent reduction in adolescent suicide rates in both Britain and the USA, although it may be starting to rise again in the USA.[70] On the other hand, there appears to be an increase in self-harm as measured by both hospital and community data. Furthermore, although the percentage of young people who report suicidal thinking is reducing, the proportion of those who also make suicidal plans is increasing.

Two possible conclusions could be drawn from these data. First, it is possible that the increase in the rate of self-harm, especially in the community, may have occurred in a population of young people who are less likely to commit suicide. Whereas the reduction in the suicide rate was mirrored by that in suicidal ideation, it was not accompanied by reduction in self-harm. Second, it is possible that young people who self-harm may be more likely to seek help than they used to, or perhaps that detection and referrals have improved. Finally, it is possible that a change in the function of self-harm has occurred. It may have acquired a different social meaning for young people and they may now be using self-harm more for the purpose of emotional regulation. The last of these possible conclusions could have the greatest implications for further research into the aetiology and treatment of self-harm.

References

1. de Wilde EJ, Kienhorst I. Suicide attempts in adolescence – 'self-report' and 'other-report'. *Crisis* 1995;16(2):59–62.
2. Hawton K, James A. Suicide and deliberate self-harm in young people. *BMJ* 2005;330(7496):891–4.
3. Evans E, Hawton K, Rodham K, Deeks J. The prevalence of suicidal phenomena in adolescents: a systematic review of population-based studies. *Suicide Life Threat Behav* 2005 Jun;35(3):239–50.
4. Hilt LM, Nock MK, Lloyd-Richardson EE, Prinstein MJ. Longitudinal study of nonsuicidal self-injury among young adolescents: rates, correlates, and preliminary test of an interpersonal model. *J Early Adolesc* 2008;28(3):455–69.
5. Briere J, Gil E. Self-mutilation in clinical and general population samples: Prevalence, correlates, and functions. *Am J Orthopsychiatry* 1998;68(4):609–20.
6. Nock MK, Prinstein MJ. A functional approach to the assessment of self-mutilative behavior. *J Consult Clin Psychol* 2004;72(5):885–90.
7. Ystgaard M, Reinholdt NP, Husby J, *et al. Tidsskr Nor Laegeforen* [Deliberate self-harm in adolescents] [English abstract] 2003;123(16):2241–5.
8. Bjarehed J, Lundh LG. Deliberate self-harm in 14-year-old adolescents: how frequent is it,

and how is it associated with psychopathology, relationship variables, and styles of emotional regulation? *Cogn Behav Ther* 2008;37(1):26–37.

9. Linehan MM, Comtois KA, Brown MZ, *et al.* Suicide attempt self-injury interview (SASII): development, reliability, and validity of a scale to assess suicide attempts and intentional self-injury. *Psychol Assess* 2006;18(3):303–12.

10. Nock MK, Holmberg EB, Photos VI, *et al.* Self-injurious thoughts and behaviors interview: development, reliability, and validity in an adolescent sample. *Psychol Assess* 2007;19(3):309–17.

11. Reynolds WM. Development of a semistructured clinical interview for suicidal behaviors in adolescents. Psychological assessment. *J Consult Clin Psychol* 1990;2(4):382–90.

12. Kaufman J, Birmaher B, Brent D, Rao U, *et al.* Schedule for affective disorders and schizophrenia for school-age children-present and lifetime version (K-SADS-PL): initial reliability and validity data. *J Am Acad Child Adolesc Psychiatry* 1997;36(7):980–8.

13. Goodman R, Ford T, Richards H, *et al.* The development and well-being assessment: description and initial validation of an integrated assessment of child and adolescent psychopathology. *J Child Psychol Psychiatry* 2000;41(5):645–55.

14. Ford T, Goodman R, Meltzer H, *et al.* The British Child and Adolescent Mental Health Survey 1999: the prevalence of DSM-IV disorders. *J Am Acad Child Adolesc Psychiatry* 2003;42(10):1203–11.

15. Shaffer D, Fisher P, Lucas CP, *et al.* NIMH Diagnostic Interview Schedule for Children Version IV (NIMH DISC-IV): description, differences from previous versions, and reliability of some common diagnoses. *J Am Acad Child Adolesc Psychiatry* 2000;39(1):28–38.

16. Reich W. Diagnostic interview for children and adolescents (DICA). *J Am Acad Child Adolesc Psychiatry* 2000;39(1):59–66.

17. Angold A, Costello EJ. The Child and Adolescent Psychiatric Assessment (CAPA). *J Am Acad Child Adolesc Psychiatry* 2000;39(1):39–48.

18. Rotheram MJ. Evaluation of imminent danger for suicide among youth. *Am J Orthopsychiatry*.1987;57(1):102–10.

19. Evans J, Evans M, Morgan HG, *et al.* Crisis card following: 12-month follow-up of a randomised controlled trial. *Br J Psychiatry* 2005;187:186–7.

20. Angold A, Costello AJ, Messer SC, *et al.* The development of a short questionnaire for use in epidemiological studies of depression in children and adolescents. *Int J Methods Psychiatr Res* 1995;5:237–49.

21. Achenbach T. *Integrative guide for the 1991 CBCL/4–18, YSR, & TRF profiles.* Burlington, VT: University of Vermont, Department of Psychiatry; 1991.

22. Achenbach T, Rescorla LA. *Manual for the ASEBA school-age forms & profiles.* Burlington, VT: University of Vermont, Research Center for Children, Youth, and Families; 2001.

23. CDC. 2009 State and Local Youth Risk Behavior Survey. Centers for Disease Control and Prevention; 2008 [accessed 20 December 2008] Available from: http://www.cdc.gov/HealthyYouth/yrbs/pdf/questionnaire/2009HighSchool.pdf.

24. Madge N, Hewitt A, Hawton K, *et al.* Deliberate self-harm within an international community sample of young people: comparative findings from the Child & Adolescent in Europe (CASE) Study. *J Child Psychol Psychiatry* 2008;49(6):667–77.

25. Addis M, Linehan MM. *Predicting suicidal behavior: psychometric properties of the Suicidal Behaviors Questionnaire.* Annual Meeting of the Association for the Advancement of Behavior Therapy; Washington, DC, 1989.

26. Harkavy Friedman JM, Asnis GM. Assessment of suicidal behavior: a new instrument. *Psychiatr Ann* 1989;**19**(7):382–7.
27. Gratz KL. Measurement of deliberate self-harm: preliminary data on the deliberate inventory. *J Psychopathol Behav Assess* 2001;**23**(4):253–63.
28. Ross S, Heath N. A study of the frequency of self-mutilation in a community sample of adolescents. *J Youth Adolesc* 2002;**31**(1):67–77.
29. Lloyd-Richardson EE, Perrine N, Dierker L, Kelley ML. Characteristic and functions on non-suicidal self-injury in a community sample of adolescents. *Psychol Med* 2007;**37**(8):1183–92.
30. Yates TM, Tracy AJ, Luthar SS. Nonsuicidal self-injury among 'privileged' youths: Longitudinal and cross-sectional approaches to developmental process. *J Consult Clin Psychol* 2008;**76**(1):52–62.
31. Gutierrez PM, Osman A, Barrios FX, Kopper BA. Development and initial validation of the Behavior Questionnaire. *J Pers Assess* 2001;**77**(3):475–90.
32. Muehlenkamp JJ, Gutierrez PM. Risk for suicide attempts among adolescents who engage in non-suicidal self-injury. *Arch Suicide Res* 2007;**11**(1):69–82.
33. McKenzie K, Bhui K, Nanchahal K, *et al.* Suicide rates in people of South Asian origin in England and Wales: 1993–2003. *Br J Psychiatry* 2008;**193**(5):406–9.
34. Neeleman J, Wessely S. Ethnic minority suicide: a small area geographical study in south London. *Psychol Med* 1999;**29**(2):429–36.
35. Matsumoto T, Imamura F, Matsumoto T, Imamura F. Self-injury in Japanese junior and senior high-school students: Prevalence and association with substance use. *Psychiatry Clin Neurosci* 2008;**62**(1):123–5.
36. Nixon MKMD, Cloutier PMA, Jansson SMP. Nonsuicidal in youth: a population-based survey. *CMAJ* 2008, **178**(3):306–12.
37. Laukkanen E, Rissanen ML, Honkalampi K, *et al.* The prevalence of self-cutting and other self-harm among 13- to 18-year-old Finnish adolescents. *Soc Psychiatry Psychiatr Epidemiol* 2009;**44**(1):23–8.
38. Nock MK, Kessler RC. Prevalence of and risk factors for suicide attempts versus suicide gestures: analysis of the National Comorbidity Survey. *J Abnorm Psychol* 2006;**115**(3):616–23.
39. Nock MK, Joiner TE, Jr, Gordon KH, *et al.* Non-suicidal self-injury among adolescents: diagnostic correlates and relation to suicide attempts. *Psychiatry Res* 2006;**144**(1):65–72.
40. Aichhorn W, Santeler S, Stelzig-Scholer R, *et al.* [Prevalence of psychiatric disorders among homeless adolescents]. *Neuropsychiatry* 2008;**22**(3):180–8.
41. Young R, Sweeting H, West P, *et al.* Prevalence of deliberate self-harm and attempted suicide within contemporary Goth youth subculture: longitudinal cohort study. *BMJ* 2006;**332**(7549):1058–61.
42. King M, Semlyen J, Tai SS, *et al.* A systematic review of mental disorder, suicide, and deliberate self-harm in lesbian, gay and bisexual people. *BMC Psychiatry* 2008;**8**:70.
43. Penn JV, Esposito CL, Schaeffer LE, *et al.* Suicide attempts and self-mutilative behavior in a juvenile correctional facility. *J Am Acad Child Adolesc Psychiatry* 2003;**42**(7):762–9.
44. Laye-Gindhu A, Schonert-Reichl KA. Nonsuicidal self-harm among community adolescents: understanding the 'Whats' and 'Whys' of self-harm. *J Youth Adolesc* 2005;**34**(5):447–57.
45. Muehlenkamp JJ, Gutierrez PM. An investigation of differences between self-injurious behavior and suicide attempts in a sample of adolescents. *Suicide Life Threat Behav* 2004;**34**(1):12–23.

46. Zoroglu SS, Tuzun U, Sar V, *et al.* Suicide attempt and self-mutilation among Turkish high school students in relation with abuse, neglect and dissociation. *Psychiatry Clin Neurosci* 2003;57(1):119–26.

47. Garrison CZ, Addy CL, McKeown RE, *et al.* Nonsuicidal physically self-damaging acts in adolescents. *J Child Fam Stud* 1993;2(4):339–52.

48. Patton GC, Harris R, Carlin J, *et al.* Adolescent suicidal behaviours: A population-based study of risk. *Psychol Med* 1997;27(3):715–24.

49. Whitlock J, Knox KL, Whitlock J, Knox KL. The relationship between self-injurious behavior and suicide in a young adult population. *Arch Pediatr Adolesc Med* 2007;161(7):634–40.

50. Walsh BW. *Treating self-injury: a practical guide*. New York, NY: Guilford Press; 2006.

51. CDC. *WISQARS Nonfatal Injury Reports*. Centers for Disease Control and Prevention 2008 [accessed 20 December 2008] Available from: http://www.cdc.gov/ncipc/wisqars/ nonfatal/definitions.htm#.

52. CDC. *WISQARS Nonfatal Injury Reports*. Centers for Disease Control and Prevention 2007 [accessed 20 December 2008] Available from: http://webappa.cdc.gov/sasweb/ncipc/ nfirates2001.html.

53. Hawton K, Casey D, Bale E, Shepherd A, Bergen H, Simkin S. Deliberate Self-harm in Oxford 2006. University of Oxford; 2006 [accessed 20 December 2008] Available from: http://cebmh.warne.ox.ac.uk/csr/images/annualreport2006.pdf.

54. Bridge JA, Goldstein TR, Brent DA. Adolescent suicide and suicidal behavior. *J Child Psychol Psychiatry* 2006;47(3,4):372–94.

55. Hawton K, Harriss L, Deliberate self-harm in young people: characteristics and subsequent mortality in a 20-year cohort of patients presenting to hospital. *J Clin Psychiatry* 2007;68(10): 1574–83.

56. Hawton K, Harriss L. Deliberate self-harm by under-15-year-olds: Characteristics, trends and outcome. *J Child Psychol Psychiatry* 2008;49(4):441–8.

57. Fergusson DM, Horwood L, Ridder EM, Beautrais AL. Suicidal behaviour in adolescence and subsequent mental health outcomes in young adulthood. *Psychol Med* 2005;35(7):983–93.

58. Steinhausen H-C, Bosiger R, Metzke CW. Stability, correlates, and outcome of adolescent suicidal risk. *J Child Psychol Psychiatry* 2006;47(7):713–22.

59. Jacobson CM, Gould M, Jacobson CM, Gould M. The epidemiology and phenomenology of non-suicidal self-injurious behavior among adolescents: a critical review of the literature. *Arch Suicide Res* 2007;11(2):129–47.

60. Eaton DK, Kann L, Kinchen S, *et al.* Youth risk behavior Surveillance United States, 2007 [accessed 20 December 2008] Available from: http://www.cdc.gov/mmwr/preview/ mmwrhtml/ss5704a1.htm.

61. Kolbe LJ, Kann L, Collins JL. Overview of the youth Risk Behavior surveillance system. *Public Health Rep* 1993;108(Suppl 1):2–10.

62. Tick NT, van der Ende J, Verhulst FC. Ten-year trends in self-reported emotional and behavioral problems of Dutch adolescents. *Soc Psychiatry Psychiatr Epidemiol* 2008;43(5):349–55.

63. Gratz KL. Risk factors for deliberate self-harm among female college students: The role and interaction of childhood maltreatment, emotional inexpressivity, and affect intensity/reactivity. *Am J Orthopsychiatry* 2006;76(2):238–50.

64. Gratz KL, Conrad SD, Roemer L. Risk factors for deliberate self-harm among college students. *Am J Orthopsychiatry* 2002;72(1):128–40.

65. WHO. Suicide Prevention (SUPRE) 2003 [accessed 28 January 2009] Available from: http://www.who.int/mental_health/prevention/suicide/.
66. Brent DA, Baugher M, Bridge J, *et al.* Age- and sex-related risk factors for adolescent suicide. *J Am Acad Child Adolesc Psychiatry* 1999;38(12):1497–505.
67. Shaffer D, Gould MS, Fisher P, *et al.* Psychiatric diagnosis in child and adolescent suicide. *Arch Gen Psychiatry* 1996;53(4):339–48.
68. Phillips MR, Li X, Zhang Y, *et al.* Suicide rates in China, 1995–99.[erratum appears in *Lancet* 2002;360(9329):344] *Lancet* 20029;359(9309):835–40.
69. Windfuhr K, While D, Hunt I, *et al.* Suicide in juveniles and adolescents in the United Kingdom. *J Child Psychol Psychiatry* 2008;49(11):1155–65.
70. Bridge JA, Greenhouse JB, Weldon AH, *et al.* Suicide trends among youths aged 10 to 19 Years in the United States, 1996–2005. *JAMA* 2008;300(9):1025–6.

CHAPTER 3

THE GENETICS OF SUICIDAL BEHAVIOUR

Colin Campbell

Introduction

A number of environmental factors have been identified which increase vulnerability to, or which precipitate, suicidal behaviour. It has been equally clear for some time that suicidal behaviour tends to aggregate within families. One plausible explanation for these observations is that environmental risk factors for suicidal behaviour, such as adverse rearing environments or childhood abuse, may be transmitted between generations. However, evidence from family, twin and adoption studies indicates that the transmission of suicidal behaviour within families is partly genetic and, to some extent, independent of the familial transmission of psychiatric disorders.

A simple way of describing the extent to which genetic factors account for the variation in a specific behaviour, or phenotype, is to determine its heritability. This is the proportion of phenotypic variance that is attributable to genetic factors in a particular population. Estimates of the heritability of suicidal behaviour derived from population-based epidemiological studies range from 30 per cent to 55 per cent. Heritability of the more narrowly defined phenotype of suicide based on register-based twin studies is estimated between 21 per cent and 51 per cent.[1]

Understanding the genetic contribution to suicidal behaviour is important as it may help identify biochemical pathways involved in the aetiology of such behaviour, which may in turn facilitate the development of more effective preventative interventions.

Recent advances in molecular genetics have provided the technology to identify susceptibility genes for specific behaviours or disorders. Initial attempts to identify genes involved in suicidal behaviour have used linkage studies or evaluated specific single nucleotide polymorphisms (SNPs) in candidate association studies.

Candidate genes for association studies have generally been selected on the basis of evidence from neurobiological and clinical studies of suicidal behaviour. The most consistently implicated neurotransmitter system is the serotonergic system. Neurobiological studies have also suggested a role for the dopaminergic and noradrenergic systems, neurotrophins and genes related to the hypothalamic–pituitary–adrenal (HPA) axis.

Genetic epidemiology

Quantitative genetic studies are designed to establish whether or not genetic factors contribute to the aetiology of a particular phenotype and, if so, what their contribution is relative to environmental factors. This is achieved by examining the extent to which various classes of relatives, who differ in how closely they are related to the index case and the degree to which they have shared a similar environment, resemble each other with respect to the phenotype in question.

Family studies

Family studies investigate the degree to which a particular behaviour or disorder aggregates within families. Familial clustering is indicated by a significantly higher risk of the relevant behaviour in relatives of probands than in control subjects. Family studies have consistently shown that suicidal behaviour aggregates within families, irrespective of variations in methodology. A meta-analysis based on findings from 21 family studies found an almost threefold greater relative risk of suicidal behaviour among close relatives of suicidal individuals thank in close relatives of non-suicidal control subjects, irrespective of psychiatric history.[2] Studies using this design have indicated that the range of suicidal behaviour, which is transmitted within families, includes suicide attempts and completions, as attempts are increased in families of completers and completed suicide is more common in families of attempters. In contrast, the familial transmission of suicidal ideation may be explained by increased familial rates of psychiatric disorder.[3,4]

Twin studies

The findings from family studies do not necessarily prove a genetic basis for suicidal behaviour as the greater risk seen in close relatives may be purely due to shared environmental factors. One method of disentangling risk attributable to shared environment from specifically genetic factors is to use twin studies. The basic premise of twin studies is that if pairs of monozygotic twins, who share 100 per cent of their genes, are more similar for a particular phenotype than pairs of dizygotic twins, who on average share 50 per cent of their genes, a genetic contribution to the phenotype can be inferred. In a replication of their previous findings, Roy and Segal[5] reviewed 28 twin pairs, in 27 of which one twin had committed suicide, and one pair in which both twins had committed suicide. The concordance for suicide in monozygotic twins was 14.9 per cent compared with 0.7 per cent in dizygotic twins. In a meta-analysis derived from seven twin studies, the relative risk of suicide attempts or completed suicide was 175 times higher in monozygotic twins than in dizygotic twins.[2] However, the authors pointed out that, because of the low incidence of suicidal behaviour in dizygotic twins included in the study, this risk ratio was probably unreliable. Some twin studies have also demonstrated the heritability of suicidal behaviour even after controlling for the effects of psychiatric disorders.[6]

Adoption studies

Another, less commonly used, method to separate shared environmental from genetic factors is adoption studies. In adoption studies the proband may be either the adoptee or the biological parent. The premise is that if the risk of the disorder is higher in biological relatives of probands (where genes are shared but not environments) than in the other control groups, a genetic contribution to the disorder is suggested. There have been relatively few adoption studies looking at suicidal behaviour and all have been based on Danish adoption records. In one study, the risk of suicidal behaviour was compared in the biological and adoptive relatives of adoptees who had committed suicide and in the biological and adoptive relatives of unaffected adoptees (who formed the control group). They found a sixfold greater suicide rate in biological relatives of adoptees who had committed suicide than in control adoptees.[7] As with those from twins studies, these findings indicate that the familial aggregation of suicidal behaviour is, in part, explained by genetic factors.

Molecular genetics of suicidal behaviour

More recently, evidence from adoption, twin and family studies has informed molecular studies, which have looked for specific genes implicated in the aetiology of suicidal behaviour. Candidate-based association studies have been the most commonly used approach thus far. In this approach, genes are selected on the basis that they affect biological systems that have been implicated in clinical or neurobiological studies and the extent to which they are associated with the phenotype in question is assessed.

Serotonergic system

The serotonergic system is the most extensively investigated neurotransmitter system in relation to suicidal behaviour. This is largely because of its role in processes central to suicidal behaviour, such as impulse control and emotional processing. Neurobiological studies have also indicated reduced central serotonergic activity in those with a history of suicidal behaviour. There is evidence of reduced cerebrospinal fluid levels of the serotonergic metabolite 5-hydroxyindole acetic acid (5-HIAA) in individuals who have attempted suicide.[8] Endocrine challenge tests of the central serotonergic system using serotonergic agonists show a blunted prolactin response in depressed patients who have attempted suicide compared with depressed patients with no such history and healthy control subjects.[9] There is also evidence of altered binding and density of serotonin receptors in the prefrontal cortex and hippocampus of suicide victims.[10]

Serotonegic genes involved in synthesis, transmission, transport and breakdown of serotonin have been investigated using association studies.

Serotonin transporter

The serotonin transporter is responsible for the re-uptake of released serotonin from the synaptic cleft. The promoter region of the gene contains a functional 44 base pair insertion/deletion variant with two common alleles, short (s) and long (l). 5-HTT transcription and serotonin re-uptake are highest in individuals homozygous for the l allele. A meta-analysis of 12 studies which pooled 1168 cases and 1371 controls found a significant association of the s allele and suicide attempts but not with completed suicide.[11] In a subsequent meta-analysis of 39 studies, the association between the 5-HTT and suicidal behaviour was confirmed using data derived from both European and Asian populations.[12]

A significant association has also been observed between a VNTR (variable number tandem repeat) polymorphism in intron 2 of the 5-HTT gene and suicide completion in patients with depression[13] and suicide attempts in patients with schizophrenia.[14]

However, the findings are by no means consistent and almost half of all association studies have found no association between these two polymorphisms and suicide across diverse populations.

Serotonin receptors

Although the common C-1019G SNP in the promoter region of the 5-HT1A receptor was found to be more common in suicide victims than in healthy control subjects[15], this association was not supported using the transmission disequilibrium test in a sample of 272 suicide attempter families.[16] Support for the role of the 5-HT1B receptor in suicidal behaviour is similarly limited. One study found an association between a SNP and a history of suicide attempts[17] but all others studies found no such association.

Increased density of 5-HT2A receptor binding sites has been described in the prefrontal cortex of suicide victims.[10] Most genetic studies have examined the common C102T SNP. A meta-analysis pooling nine studies found no association between the C102T SNP and suicidal behaviour.[11] A subsequent meta-analysis based on 25 studies also failed to find an association with C102T but found a significant role for the A1438G polymorphism.[18] Given the number of negative studies, further investigation of the role of the 5-HT2A receptor is needed.

No significant association has been found between suicidal behaviour and the 5-HT1D, 5-HT1E, 5-HT1F, 5-HT2C, 5-HT5A and 5-HT6 receptors and some of the 12 known 5-HT receptor subtypes have yet to be investigated.

Tryptophan hydroxylase

Tryptophan hydroxylase catalyses the initial and rate-limiting step in the synthesis of serotonin. Despite extensive investigation, individual studies and metanalyses investigating the role of the TPH1 gene and suicidal behaviour have produced conflicting results. An early meta-analysis failed to find an association between the A218C SNP in intron 7 of TPH1 and suicidal behaviour. A subsequent meta-analysis based on 22 studies confirmed a strong association between the A218C and A779C polymorphisms and suicidal behaviour[19]. The genetic analysis of this gene has been complicated further by the discovery of the TPH2 gene. TPH1 is mainly expressed in the periphery, whereas TPH2 is preferentially expressed in the brainstem. A number of variants in the TPH2 gene have been identified and used as markers in association studies. Homozygotes for the T allele of SNP rs4448371 and the G allele of SNP rs4641527 were more common among depressed patients who had committed suicide than those who had not.[20] Several studies have failed to find any associations between TPH2 variants and suicidal behaviour and further studies are needed to clarify the role of this gene in suicidal behaviour.

Monoamine oxidase A

Monoamine oxidase A (MAOA) is responsible for the deamination of bioamines, such as serotonin and noradrenaline. Most studies have focused on a VNTR polymorphism in the promoter region, which has been associated with violent suicide attempts in men.[21] This finding was supported by Ho and colleagues,[22] who reported an association between the VNTR polymorphism and suicide attempts in patients with bipolar affective disorder. They also found an association between the Fnu4H1 polymorphism and suicide attempts but in female patients only. Despite these positive findings, a number of studies have failed to find any significant differences in genotype of allele distribution between individuals with suicidal behaviour and control subjects.

Noradrenergic and dopaminergic systems

Although less extensively investigated than the serotonergic system, the noradrenergic and dopaminergic systems have a role in a number of processes related to suicidal behaviour, such as response to stress, and are therefore good candidates for molecular genetic studies. Neurobiological studies have also implicated these neurotransmitter systems in suicidal behaviour. There is evidence that there are fewer noradrenergic neurons[23] and increased alpha-2-adrenoceptor agonist binding in the locus coeruleus of suicide victims.[24] Some studies have indicated that levels of the dopamine metabolite, HMVA, in the cerebrospinal fluid (CSF) are negatively correlated with suicidal behaviour, although this finding has not been consistently replicated.[25] Depressed patients with a history of suicide attempts have also been shown to have a blunted growth hormone response to the dopaminergic agonist apomorphine.[26]

Tyrosine hydroxylase

Tyrosine hydroxylase (TH) is the rate-limiting enzyme in the synthesis of catecholamines, including noradrenaline and dopamine. Although immunoreactivity of TH has been reported to be reduced in the locus coeruleus of individuals who have completed suicide,[27] some studies have failed to replicate this finding. The Th-K3 allele of the TH gene is associated with suicide attempts in patients with adjustment disorders and there is a tendency for a low incidence of the TH-K1 allele among suicide attempters.[28] Significantly lower levels of 3-methoxy, 4-hydroxy phenyl glycol (MHPG, the main metabolite of noradrenaline) have been described in Th-K3 allele carriers.[29]

Catechol-O-methyl transferase

Catechol-O-methyl transferase (COMT) is the main enzyme involved in the inactivation of noradrenaline and dopamine. There is a common Val158Met polymorphism and 158Val homozygotes have three to four times the enzyme activity of Met homozygotes. A positive association has been reported between the low-activity 158Met allele and violent suicide attempts in men with schizophrenia or schizoaffective disorder[30]. However, the evidence regarding the role of COMT in suicidal behaviour is inconsistent and some studies have failed to find an association between suicidal behaviour and COMT genotype frequencies[31].

Dopamine D2 receptor

A SNP in the 3´-untranslated region of exon 8 (E8) of the DRD2 gene has been associated with suicidal behaviour. The frequent E8 A/A genotype was associated with increased suicide attempts, depression and anxiety scores in patients with alcohol dependence.[32] Johann and colleagues[33] found the –141C deletion allele of the –141C insertion/deletion polymorphism to be over-represented in patients with alcohol dependence with a history of suicidality. However, another study found no association between the –141C insertion/deletion polymorphism and suicidal behaviour in a sample of patients with depressive disorders.[22]

Alpha-2A-adrenergic receptor

Genetic variation in four loci in the alpha-2A-adrenergic receptor gene were investigated in a sample of suicide victims and in control subjects. The three loci in the promoter region showed no difference in allelic or genotypic expression between suicide victims and control subjects. The rare 251K allele of the fourth potentially functional locus, N251K, was only found in suicide cases.[34]

Neurotrophic factors

Neurotrophins are a family of small proteins secreted in the nervous system that control the survival, differentiation and growth of neurons.

Brain-derived neurotrophic factor

Brain-derived neurotrophic factor (BDNF) is the most abundant neurotrophic factor in the brain. Reduced BDNF mRNA has been reported in the prefrontal cortex and the hippocampus of individuals who completed suicide.[35] Perroud and colleagues[36] investigated whether the Val66Met BDNF polymorphism moderated the effect of childhood maltreatment on suicidal behaviour. Childhood sexual abuse was associated with an increased risk of violent suicide only in Val/Val individuals and not in Val/Met or Met/Met individuals.

Low-affinity neurotrophin receptor p75^{NTR}

The minor (L205) allele of the common missense polymorphism (S205L) of the gene coding for p75^{NTR} was found to be significantly decreased in patients with depressive disorder compared with control subjects, particularly in those with a history of suicide attempts.[37]

Other factors

Corticotrophin-releasing hormone receptor 1 (CRHR1)

Genes involved in the HPA axis are important candidates, as altered HPA axis activity may be related to the risk of suicidal behaviour. One study reported an association between an SNP in the CRH receptor gene (rs4792887) and suicide attempt in depressed men exposed to low lifetime levels of stress, but not in those with high stress levels.[38]

GABA$_A$ receptor

Reduced mRNA coding for the α1, α3, α4 and δsubunits of the GABA$_A$ receptor has been reported in the frontopolar regions of individuals who have completed suicide.[39] However, no relationship was found between four frequent variants (A1, A2, A3 and A4) of the α3 subunit and suicide attempts.[40]

Angiotensin-converting enzyme

In addition to its role in the rennin–angiotensin system, angiotensin II also has a role in the brain, where it degrades substance P. Substance P has been implicated in the aetiology of depression and may regulate the serotonergic system in the dorsal raphe nuclei. The I allele of the ACEI/D polymorphism has been shown to be significantly more frequent in individuals who completed suicide than in control subjects.[41]

Gene–gene and gene–environment interactions

Although preliminary and at times inconsistent, the available evidence points to a role for both genetic and environmental factors in the aetiology of suicidal behaviour. These factors may interact additively, that is the risk attributable to genetic factors is added to that which comes from environmental experiences, resulting in an overall liability to develop suicidal behaviour. However, another possibility is that risk factors may interact in ways that exceed additive and linear effects.

Genetic factors may interact with each other so that the effects of one gene on the phenotype of interest may be masked or enhanced by one or more other genes. They may also interact with environmental factors by influencing sensitivity and exposure to particular environmental stressors.

Evidence for the latter type of interaction has been described where a functional polymorphism in the 5-HTT gene was found to moderate the influence of stressful life events on depression and suicidality in a birth cohort. The gene–environment interaction showed that stressful life events predicted a diagnosis of depression, suicidal ideation and suicide attempts among carriers of an s allele but not among l/l homozygotes.[42]

Future work

The evidence thus far indicates that suicidal behaviour is a multifactorial phenotype with several genes exerting a small effect moderated by interaction with numerous environmental factors. The data thus far are often inconsistent and the field is characterised by a lack of replication of findings. This could be addressed in future research in a number of ways.

The definition of the phenotype often varies between studies, from suicidal ideation to completed suicide. This can result in inconsistent findings and failure to replicate findings, particularly when large numbers of genes, each with a small effect, are contributing to the phenotype. A narrower definition of the suicidal behaviour phenotype may make small gene effects easier to detect, as could controlling for known moderators, such as gender or ethnicity. This might also increase the currently limited understanding of the role of genetic factors in non-suicidal self-injurious behaviour, as existing studies rarely distinguish between suicidal and non-suicidal self-injury.[43]

This issue could also be addressed by looking for associations with intermediate phenotypes, or endophenotypes, such as impulsive aggression or cognitive function, which may be more specifically defined and measured. Endophenotypes may be easier to detect as they are more proximal to genetic factors. They may also be helpful in elucidating the neurobiological mechanisms involved and the intermediate steps between gene expression and behaviour.

Future studies could also include examination of known environmental risk factors and establish the nature and extent of their interaction with the genetic factor of interest. This might go some way to explain the often inconsistent findings and highlight the developmental differences in the correlations seen between specific risk factors and suicidal behaviour.

Although the candidate association approach has been successful in identifying some genes which may have a role in the aetiology of suicidal behaviour, a more systematic approach to identifying functional polymorphisms would be helpful as it may identify genes not implicated by clinical or neurobiological studies but which may play a more direct role in susceptibility to suicidal behaviour. Achieving this task has been made more feasible by the development of microarray technology, which can be employed to profile the expression of thousands of genes simultaneously.

Summary

Evidence from adoption, twin and family studies supports the notion that the aetiology of suicidal behaviour is partly genetic. Guided by the findings from these studies and neurobiological research on suicidal behaviour, a number of genes have been identified using the candidate gene approach. The serotonergic system is the most consistently implicated neurotransmitter system in suicidal behaviour and some of the findings relating to serotonergic genes have been reasonably well replicated, e.g. 5-HTT. Findings for other candidate genes have been less consistent and further work is required to understand the role of these genes in the aetiology of suicidal behaviour. Future work should be based on a refined phenotype, or possibly endophenotypes, and should attempt to identify possible gene–gene and gene–environment interactions.

References

1. Voracek M, Loibl LM. Genetics of suicide: a systematic review of twin studies. *Wein Klin Wochenschr* 2007;119:463–75.
2. Baldessarini RJ, Hennen J. Genetics of suicide: an overview. *Harv Rev Psychiatry* 2004;12:1–13.
3. Brent DA, Bridge J, Johnson BA, Connolly J. Suicidal behaviour runs in families. A controlled family study of adolescent suicide victims. *Arch Gen Psychiatry* 1996;53: 1145–52.
4. Brent DA, Melhem N. Familial transmission of suicidal behaviour. *Psychiatr Clin North Am* 2008;319(2):157–77.
5. Roy A, Segal NL. Suicidal behaviour in twins: a replication. *J Affect Disord* 2001;66:71–4.
6. Fu Q, Heath AC, Bucholz KK, *et al.* A twin study of genetic and environmental influences on suicidality in men. *Psychol Med* 2002;32:11–24.
7. Schlusinger F, Key SS, Rosenthal D, Wender PH. A family study of suicide. In: Schou M, Stromgren E, editors. *Origin, prevention and treatment of affective disorders*. London: Academic Press; 1979: pp. 277–87.
8. Åsberg M. Neurotransmitters and suicidal behaviour. The evidence from cerebrospinal fluid studies. *Ann N Y Acad Sci* 1997;836:158–81.
9. Corrêa H, Duval F, Mokrani M, *et al.* Prolactin response to D-fenfluramine and suicidal behaviour in depressed patients. *Psychiatry Res* 2000;93:189–99.
10. Pandey GN, Dwivedi Y, Rizavi HS, *et al.* Higher expression of serotonin 5-HT2A receptors in the brains of teenage suicide victims. *Am J Psychiatry* 2002;159:419–29.
11. Anguelova M, Benkelfat C, Turecki G. A systematic review of association studies

investigating genes coding for serotonin receptors and the serotonin transporter: II Suicidal behaviour. *Mol Psychiatry* 2003;8:646–53.

12. Li D, He L. Meta-analysis supports association between serotonin transporter (5-HTT) and suicidal behaviour. *Mol Psychiatry* 2007;12:47–54.

13. Lopez de Lara C, Dumais A, Rouleau G, *et al.* STin2 variant and family history of suicide as significant predictors of suicide completion in major depression. *Biol Psychiatry* 2006;59:114–20.

14. De Luca V, Zai G, Tharmalingam S, *et al.* Association study between the novel functional polymorphism of the serotonin transporter gene and suicidal behaviour in schizophrenia. *Eur Neuropsychopharmacol* 2006;16:268–71.

15. Lemonde S, Turecki G, Bakish D, *et al.* Impaired repression at a 5-hydroxytryptamine 1A receptor gene polymorphism associated with major depression and suicide. *J Neurosci* 2003;23:8788–99.

16. Wasserman D, Geijer T, Sokolowski M, *et al.* The serotonin 1A receptor C(−1019)G polymorphism in relation to suicide attempt. *Behav Brain Funct* 2006;2:14.

17. New AS, Gelernter J, Goodman M, *et al.* Suicide, impulsive aggression and HTR1B genotype. *Biol Psychiatry* 2001;50:62–5.

18. Li D, Duan Y, He L. Association study of serotonin receptor (5-HT2A) gene with schizophrenia and suicidal behaviour using systematic meta-analysis. *Biochem Biophys Res Commun* 2006;340:1006–16.

19. Li D, He L. Further clarification of the contribution of the tryptophan hydroxylase (TPH) gene to suicidal behaviour using systematic allelic and genotypic meta-analyses. *Hum Genet* 2006;119:233–40.

20. Lopez de Lara C, Brezo J, Rouleau G, *et al.* Effect of tryptophan hydroxylase-2 gene variants on suicide risk in major depression. *Biol Psychiatry* 2007;62:72–80.

21. Courtet P, Jollant F, Buresi C, *et al.* The monoamine oxidase A gene may influence the means used in suicide attempts. *Psychiatr Genet* 2005;15:189–93.

22. Ho LW, Furlong RA, Rubinsztein JS, *et al.* Genetic associations with clinical characteristics in bipolar affective disorder and recurrent unipolar affective disorder. *Am Journal Med Genet* 2000;96:36–42.

23. Arango V, Underwood MD, Mann JJ. Fewer pigmented locus coeruleus neurons in suicide victims: preliminary results. *Biol Psychiatry* 1996;39:112–20.

24. Ordway GA, Widdowson PS, Smith KS, Halaris A. Agonist binding to alpha 2-adrenoreceptors is elevated in the locus coeruleus from victims of suicide. *J Neurochem* 1994;63:617–24.

25. Placidi GP, Oquendo MA, Malone KM, *et al.* Aggressivity, suicide attempts, and depression: relationships to cerebrospinal fluid monoamine metabolite levels. *Biol Psychiatry* 2001;50:783–91.

26. Pitchot W, Hansenne M, Ansseau M. Suicidal behaviour and growth hormone response to apomorphine test. *Biol Psychiatry* 1992;31:121–19.

27. Biegon A, Fieldust S. Reduced tyrosine hydroxylase immunoreactivity in locus coeruleus of suicide victims. *Synapse* 1992;10:79–82.

28. Persson ML, Wasserman D, Geijer T, *et al.* Tyrosine hydroxylase allelic distribution in suicide attempters. *Psychiatry Res* 1997;72:73–80.

29. Jönsson E, Sedvall G, Brené S, *et al.* Dopamine-related genes and their relationships to monoamine metabolites in CSF. *Biol Psychiatry* 1996;40:1032–43.

30. Nolan KA, Volavka J, Czobor P, *et al.* Suicidal behaviour in patients with schizophrenia is related to COMT polymorphism. *Psychiatr Genet*;10:117–24.

31. Russ MJ, Lachman HM, Kashdan T, *et al.* Analysis of catechol-O-methyltransferase and 5-hydroxytryptamine transporter polymorphisms in patients at risk for suicide. *Psychiatry Res* 2000;93:73–8.

32. Finckh U, Rommelspacher H, Kuhn S, *et al.* Influence of the dopamine D2 receptor (DRD2) genotype on neuroadaptive effects of alcohol and the clinical outcome of alcoholism. *Pharmacogenetics* 1997;7:271–81.

33. Johann M, Putzhammer A, Eichhammer P, Wodarz N. Association of the –141C Del variant of the dopamine D2 receptor (DRD2) with positive family history and suicidality in German alcoholics. *Am J Med Genet B NeuroPsychiatr Genet* 2005;132:46–9.

34. Sequeira A, Mamdani F, Lalovic A, *et al.* Alpha 2A adrenergic receptor gene and suicide. *Psychiatry Res* 2004;125:87–93.

35. Dwivedi Y, Rizavi HS, Conley RR, *et al.* Altered gene expression of brain-derived neurotrophic factor and receptor tyrosine kinase B in post-mortem brain of suicide subjects. *Arch Gen Psychiatry* 2003;60;804–15.

36. Perroud N, Courtet P, Vincze I, Jaussent I, *et al.* Interaction between BDNF Val66Met and childhood maltreatment on adult's violent suicide attempt. *Genes Brain Behav* 2008;7:314–22.

37. Kunugi H, Hashimoto R, Yoshida M, *et al.* A missense polymorphism (S205L) of the low-affinity neurotrophin receptor p75NTR gene is associated with depressive disorder and attempted suicide. *Am J Med Genet B NeuroPsychiatr Genet* 2004;129;44–6.

38. Wasserman D, Sokolowski M, Rozanov V, Wasserman J. The CRHR1 gene: a marker for suicidality in depressed males exposed to low stress. *Genes Brain Behav* 2008;7:14–19.

39. Merali Z, Du L, Hrdina P, *et al.* Dysregulation in the suicide brain: mRNA expression of corticotropin-releasing hormone receptors and GABA$_A$ receptor subunits in frontal cortical brain region. *J Neurosci* 2004;24:1478–85.

40. Baca-Garcia E, Vaquero C, Diaz-Sastre C, *et al.* Lack of association between polymorphic variations in the α3 subunit GABA receptor gene (GABRA3) and suicide attempts. *Prog Neuropsychopharmacol Biol Psychiatry* 2004; 28: 409–12.

41. Hishimoto A, Shirakawa O, Nishiguchi N, *et al.* Association between a functional polymorphism in the rennin-angiotensin system and completed suicide. *J Neural Transm* 2006;113:1915–20.

42. Caspi A, Sugden K, Moffitt TE, *et al.* Influence of life stress on depression: moderation by a polymorphism in the 5-HTT gene. *Science* 2003;301:386–9.

43. Jacobson CM, Gould M. The epidemiology and phenomenology of non-suicidal self-injurious behaviour among adolescents: a critical review of the literature. *Arch Suicide Res* 2007;11:129–47.

CHAPTER 4

THE NEUROBIOLOGY OF SELF-HARM

Elaine Chung

Introduction

The neurobiology of self-harm is a field that has been developed significantly over the past 30 years. The aims of this work include to further our understanding of the biological mechanisms of self-harm, and to introduce the possibility of developing complementary biological risk assessment strategies and future therapeutic interventions. Self-harm occurs in a number of conditions; however, there is increasing evidence for certain characteristic neurobiological findings in self-harm independent of psychiatric diagnosis. Much of the literature examines 'suicidal behaviour', (which in the USA tends to include at least some intent to end one's life, unlike in Europe),[1] while some studies more specifically examine borderline personality disorder. The majority of the literature has looked at adult populations. The neurobiology of self-harm in young people is in a more embryonic stage, despite adolescence being noted as a period of significant vulnerability with respect to neurobiological development,[2] and there being a growing literature in the developmental psychopathology of borderline personality disorder.[3] Research methods comprise the use of animal models, *in vivo* and post-mortem studies of neurotransmitters, their metabolites, receptor binding, receptor density and second messenger systems, and more recently functional neuroimaging studies. Genetic studies are also contributing significantly to knowledge of the neurobiology of self-harm and are discussed in Chapter 3. More exciting recent developments are in elucidating the clinical endophenotypes of suicidal behaviour and their relationship to neurobiological findings, thus forming psychobiological hypotheses of self-harm.

The serotonergic system

Serotonin is a catecholamine neurotransmitter. There is a large body of evidence from *in vivo* and post-mortem studies implicating serotonergic dysfunction in suicidal behaviour, independent of associated psychiatric diagnosis.[4]

Asberg et al.[5] first demonstrated the association between suicide attempts and low concentrations of the serotonin metabolite, 5-hydroxyindoleacetic acid (5-HIAA) in the cerebrospinal fluid (CSF) in 1976. Since then, this association of low CSF 5-HIAA and suicidal behaviour has been replicated in more than 20 studies across a range of diagnostic categories, including depression, schizophrenia, personality disorders, and also in violent offenders, although interestingly not in bipolar affective disorder.[6] This association is most prominent in those utilising violent methods of self-harm.[6] There is also evidence that low CSF 5-HIAA predicts future suicide attempts and completed suicide,[7] suggesting that this reflects a stable trait. Low CSF 5-HIAA is also associated with aggression and impulsivity.[8]

Neuroendocrine studies, described as the 'window to the brain',[9] provide means of investigating serotonergic function. Fenfluramine causes the release of serotonin from presynaptic storage granules and inhibits its reuptake, and the degree to which it stimulates serotonin can be measured by levels of prolactin. Serotonergic hypofunction in suicidality is also demonstrated by the blunted prolactin response following fenfluramine challenge in people with depression, and personality disorders, who have attempted suicide, compared with control subjects.[9] Decreased prolactin response is greater in high-lethality than in low-lethality suicidal attempts.[10] On functional neuroimaging utilising positron emission tomography, decreased prefrontal cortex serotonergic functioning distinguished high- from low-lethality suicide attempters.[11] New et al.[12] have also shown blunted prolactin and cortisol response to fenfluramine challenge in people with personality disorders and non-suicidal self-harm, supporting evidence for serotonergic dysfunction in both suicidal and non-suicidal self-harm. Blunted prolactin response to fefluramine challenge is also seen in impulsive and aggressive individuals.[13]

Post-mortem, and more recently functional neuroimaging studies of serotonin receptor binding and the serotonin transporter (SERT also known as 5-HTT) also support a relationship between suicidality and the serotonin system, although conflicting results may be due to methodological complications in terms of the heterogeneous distribution of receptors in the brain and differences in radioligands used for binding. Serotonin transporters are located on the axon terminals of serotonin neurons and are responsible for serotonin reuptake. SERT binding is one index of the serotonergic innervation of cortical areas. Results of SERT binding studies suggest that there is a reduction in transporter binding in the ventromedial prefrontal cortex of suicide victims.[14–16] Binding studies of the post-synaptic 5-HT2A receptor in the central nervous system also vary according to the neuroanatomical site examined; however, more studies point to an increase in 5-HT2A receptor density in the prefrontal cortex.[8,15,17] It is hypothesised that the increase in 5-HT2A receptor density is due to upregulation in response to serotonin depletion.[18] Pandey et al.[19] found that the greater numbers of 5-HT2A receptors in the prefrontal cortex and hippocampus of teenage suicide victims was also contributed to by increased gene expression. The ventral prefrontal cortex is associated with behavioural and cognitive inhibition, and it is thought that this area is part of a restraint mechanism whose function modulates the probability of suicidal behaviour and aggression. Oquendo et al.[20] found a significant correlation between lifetime aggression scores and prefrontal 5-HT2A receptor binding in subjects who had died by suicide, which was not found in those who had died by other means. In in-vivo functional neuroimaging studies, however, reduced binding potential of the 5-HT2A receptor in the dorsolateral prefrontal cortex has been shown in people who had self-harmed compared with normal control subjects, with the greatest reduction in those utilising violent means.[21] Compared with normal control subjects, people who had attempted suicide had a significantly lower binding potential of frontal 5-HT2A receptors, and this was significantly correlated with harm avoidance and hopelessness measures.[22] Platelets provide a more convenient peripheral substrate for examining serotonergic function, and potentially a minimally invasive biological marker for identifying suicidality. Platelets have many of the properties of the serotonin nerve terminal: they are embryonically derived from neural crest and contain 5-HT2A receptors, serotonin transporters and a subcellular store of serotonin.[8] While imipramine binding sites in the platelets of suicidal patients and changes in serotonin uptake have shown conflicting results, there have been consistent findings of an increase in platelet 5-HT2A in suicidal patients, independent of diagnosis.[9] Pandey[9] further found that this increase was specific to the patients with recent suicide attempts or ideation and was not found in those who had attempted suicide more than 6 months previously, suggesting that the increase in platelet 5-HT2A receptors may be state related. In studies of young people, Crowell et al.[23] found that whole blood serotonin levels were significantly lower in parasuicidal adolescent girls than in age-matched normal control subjects. Tyano et al.[24] found that plasma serotonin levels were significantly negatively correlated with suicidal behaviour severity and lower in violent than in non-violent subjects; however, the serotonin plasma concentration in the clinically referred group was higher than in healthy control subjects. Mean whole blood tryptophan (from which the amino acid serotonin is synthesised) content was significantly lower among pre-pubertal inpatients with a recent suicide attempt than in normal control subjects.[25]

There is therefore a considerable body of evidence implicating dysfunction of the serotonergic system in suicidal behaviour and this is likely to be a trait-dependent characteristic associated with disturbances in impulsivity, aggression and anxiety. The results of the studies are conflicting but overall point towards state-dependent serotonergic hypoactivity. The precise relationship between serotonin and self-harm in this age group has yet to be understood.

The noradrenergic system

Noradrenaline is a catecholamine with dual roles as a neurotransmitter and hormone and exerts its actions via binding to adrenergic receptors. While less studied than the serotonergic system, there is some evidence for a state-related hyperactivity of the noradrenergic system in suicidality.[1]

Post-mortem studies reveal fewer noradrenergic neurons in the locus coeruleus of suicide victims than in normal control subjects.[26] Noradrenaline levels are decreased in the brainstem of suicide victims, while alpha-2-adrenoceptor numbers are increased, perhaps upregulated secondary to the lower noradrenaline levels.[27] Tyrosine hydroxylase (TH) is the rate-limiting enzyme in the biosynthesis of noradrenaline, and its immunoreactivity increases as a compensatory mechanism where increased noradrenaline release leads to depletion of the neurotransmitter.[15] The findings of both increased and decreased TH immunoreactivity in suicide victims are therefore thought to provide evidence that these could be state dependent. Evidence from the pre-cortex suggests increased beta-2-adrenergic receptor binding, and increased noradrenaline levels and alpha-adrenergic binding in suicide victims. This cortical noradrenergic activity may result in depletion of noradrenaline from the smaller population of noradrenergic neurons found in suicide victims.[15] These findings suggest an association with an increased stress response before suicide, resulting in excessive noradrenaline release.[1,15]

In-vivo studies of noradrenergic function in suicidal behaviour show a relationship between reduced urinary excretion of the primary metabolite of noradrenaline, 3-methoxy, 4-hydroxy phenyl glycol (MHPG), and a past history of suicide attempts.[28] The majority of studies show no correlation of CSF MHPG with suicide.[6] There is a blunted response to challenge with the alpha-2-adrenergic agonist, clonidine, in suicide attempters, suggesting low alpha-2-adrenoreceptor activity. These findings indicate that noradrenaline dysfunction found, for example, in severe anxiety might contribute to self-harm.[15]

The hypothalamic–pituitary–adrenal axis

The hypothalamic–pituitary–adrenal (HPA) axis is the neuroendocrine system that regulates the body's responses to stress. Stress leads to the release of the corticotrophin-releasing hormone (CRH), which activates the HPA axis by stimulating the release of adrenocorticotrophin (ACTH) and hence the release of corticosteroids from the adrenal glands. The HPA axis has complex interactions with central serotonergic, noradrenergic and dopaminergic systems. Hyperactivity of the HPA axis is also implicated in suicidal behaviour.[1,15]

Elevated urinary cortisol has been found in patients with a history of violent suicidal behaviour compared with non-suicidal patients. This also correlated with personality profiles of low-reward dependence (reflecting the degree of sensitivity to social stressors) and a tendency to raised novelty-seeking scores (related to impulsivity and anger regulation) in this population.[29] Larger adrenal glands and decreased prefrontal cortical CRH binding has also been shown in suicide victims.[15,30]

The dexamethasone suppression test (DST) provides a means of measuring HPA activity. Non-suppression of cortisol release in response to administration of dexamethasone indicates hyperactivity of the HPA axis. Some, but not all studies, have found an association between dexamethasone non-suppression and suicidality. In a 15-year follow-up study, Coryell *et al.*[31] found that dexamethasone non-suppression of cortisol at baseline may be associated with a 14-fold increase in the risk of completed suicide.

In pre-pubertal children, significantly higher plasma cortisol levels at 4pm (but not those taken at other times) were found in suicidal than in non-suicidal inpatients, independent of diagnosis. The dexamethasone suppression test (DST) has not been found to distinguish suicidal pre-pubertal children from others.[32]

It is also thought that HPA overactivity may lead to, or exacerbate, the serotonin abnormalities observed in suicidal brains.[33] The corticosteroid modulation of 5-HT receptors may provide a potential mechanism for intervention in suicidal behaviours and affective disorders.[33,34]

The dopaminergic system

Dopamine is a catecholamine neurotransmitter and neurohormone. It is the precursor to noradrenaline and adrenaline and also interacts with the HPA axis. Dopaminergic system abnormalities are found in depression; however, there are too few studies to determine its association with suicide.[15] *In-vivo* studies found reduced growth hormone response to the dopaminergic agonist, apomorphine, in suicide attempters versus non-attempters, suggesting a role for the D_2 dopaminergic receptor.[35]

Dopamine deficiency is strongly implicated in self-injurious behaviours with evidence from preclinical studies in rats, and most particularly in Lesch–Nyhan syndrome.[36–38]

Opioids

There is a significant body of research in self-injurious behaviour suggesting dysregulated proopiomelanocortin (POMC) and opioid systems in which increased pain tolerance and or addiction to endogenous opioids is proposed.[37,39] There are far fewer studies of this system in suicide. However, increased μ-receptor density in the frontal cortex and caudate, but not the thalamus, has been shown in suicide victims in one study [8] and in the frontal and temporal cortical gyri of younger (<41 years) but not older suicide victims compared with age-matched control subjects.[40]

Signal transduction abnormalities in suicidal behaviour

Protein kinase C (PKC) is a critical phosphorylating enzyme in the phosphoinositide signal transduction pathway for 5-HT2A and other receptors, mediating their functional response. There is evidence for its role in mental disorders, and decreased activity of PKC has been demonstrated in the brains of teenage suicide victims compared with non-psychiatric control subjects.[41] Reduced levels of CREB, the cyclic-AMP-responsive element binding factor, its DNA binding activity and the cAMP-dependent activity of protein kinase A (PKA) are found in the hippocampus and prefrontal cortex of suicide victims.[15,42] A deficiency of selective G-protein α-subunits is also associated with suicide, independent of psychiatric diagnosis.[15,43] Therefore, the effects of receptor upregulation may be offset by impaired signal transduction in suicidality.[15] As these second messenger systems are also affected by psychoactive drugs such as lithium, they may provide a focus of therapeutic intervention.

Other neurobiological findings

There are studies investigating the role of endocannabionoids,[44] neurotrophins[45,46] and cholesterol[47,48] in self-harm and suicide; however, it is too early to draw firm conclusions about their role.

Neuroimaging findings

Abnormal fronto-limbic circuitry is implicated in studies in both borderline personality disorder and depressed, suicidal patients compared with non-suicidal depressed subjects.[49,50]

Neurobiological models of suicidal behaviour

The findings discussed above have been integrated into a number of neurobiological models of suicidal behaviour.

Kamali et al.[8] and Mann[15] propose a stress diathesis model of suicidal behaviour whereby an underlying diathesis such as a tendency towards aggression, impulsivity or hopelessness, influenced by other factors including gender, genetic factors and childhood experiences, in the context of a stressor such as an acute psychosocial crisis, combined with a psychiatric illness, could lead to suicidal behaviour. This model helps explain why one person may attempt suicide during a depressive episode, while another may not. Targeting neurobiological aspects of the diathesis may provide opportunities for therapeutic intervention.[15]

Van Heeringen's[1] process model of suicidal behaviour is also based on a state–trait interaction, and further incorporates the gradual evolution of suicidality over time. It includes three cognitive characteristics of 'defeat' (a tendency to perceive oneself as a loser when confronted with a psychosocial stressor), perceptions of 'no escape' (associated with autobiographical memory impairment and problem-solving deficits leading to perceived entrapment) and perceptions of 'no rescue' or hopelessness.

Serotonergic hypoactivity appears to be state dependent, whereas hyperactivity of the HPA axis and noradrenergic systems appears to be state related and involved in the response to stressful events.

Carballo *et al.*[34] recently proposed an integrative model of biological and clinical findings in suicidal behaviour, whereby developmental factors comprising genetic factors and psychological or clinical factors may have causal roles in the disturbances found in suicidal subjects. Genotype and early childhood experience may influence the manifestation of neurobiological (HPA axis, serotonin, noradrenaline, dopamine) and clinical endophenotypes (aggression, impulsivity, pessimism and neuroticism) associated with suicidal behaviour.

Summary

Knowledge regarding the neurobiology of suicide and self-harm, independent of psychiatric diagnoses, while still limited, is increasing and is beginning to tie together neurobiological and clinical diatheses of suicide. In future this may assist not only our growing understanding of suicidality, but also improve prevention and risk assessment and help develop improved therapeutic interventions.

References

1. Van Heeringen K. The neurobiology of suicide and suicidality. *Can J Psychiatry* 2003;48(5):292–300.
2. Dahl RE. Adolescent brain development: a period of vulnerabilities and opportunities. Keynote address. *Ann N Y Acad Sci* 2004;1021:1–22.
3. Gollan JK, Lee R, Coccaro EF. Developmental psychopathology and neurobiology of aggression. *Dev Psychopathol* 2005;17:1151–71.
4. Mann JJ, Brent MN, Arango V. The neurobiology and genetics of suicide and attempted suicide: a focus on the serotonergic system. *Neuropsychopharmacology* 2001;24(5):467–77.
5. Asberg M, Traskman L, Thoren P. 5-HIAA in the cerebrospinal fluid. A biochemical suicide predictor? *Arch Gen Psychiatry* 1976;33(10):1193–97.
6. Asberg M. Neurotransmitters and suicidal behavior. The evidence from cerebrospinal fluid studies. *Ann N Y Acad Sci* 1997;836:158–81.
7. Nordström P, Samuelsson M, Asberg M, *et al.* CSF 5-HIAA predicts suicide risk after attempted suicide. *Suicide Life Threat Behav* 1994;24(1):1–9.
8. Kamali M, Oquendo MA, Mann JJ. Understanding the neurobiology of suicidal behaviour. *Depress Anxiety* 2001;14:164–76.
9. Pandey GH. Altered serotonin function in suicide. Evidence from platelet and neuroendocrine studies. *Ann N Y Acad Sci* 1997;836:182–200.
10. Malone KM, Corbitt EM, Li S, Mann JJ. Prolactin response to fenfluramine and suicide attempt lethality in major depression. *Br J Psychiatry* 1996;168:324–9.
11. Oquendo MA, Placidi GPA, Malone KM, *et al.* Positron emission tomography of regional brain metabolic responses to a serotonergic challenge and lethality of suicide attempts in major depression. *Arch Gen Psychiatry* 2003;60:14–22.

12. New AS, Trestman RL, Mitropoulou V, *et al*. Serotonergic function and self-injurious behavior in personality disorder patients. *Psychiatry Res* 1997;69(1):17–26.

13. Coccaro EF, Siever LJ, Klar HM, *et al*. Serotonergic studies in patients with affective and personality disorders. Correlates with suicidal and impulsive aggressive behavior. *Arch Gen Psychiatry* 1989;46(7):587–99.

14. Mann JJ, Huang Y, Underwood MD, *et al*. A serotonin transporter gene promoter polymorphism (5-HTTLPR) and prefrontal cortical binding in major depression and suicide. *Arch Gen Psychiatry* 2000;57:729–38.

15. Mann JJ. Neurobiology of suicidal behaviour. *Nat Rev Neurosci* 2003;4:819–28.

16. Arango V, Underwood MD, Gubbi AV, Mann JJ. Localized alterations in pre- and postsynaptic serotonin binding sites in the ventrolateral prefrontal cortex of suicide victims. *Brain Res* 1995;688:121–33.

17. Turecki G, Brière R, Dewar K, *et al*. Prediction of level of serotonin 2_A receptor binding by serotonin receptor 2_A genetic variation in postmortem brain samples from subjects who did or did not commit suicide. *Am J Psychiatry* 1999;156:1456–8.

18. Mann JJ, Arango V, Underwood MD. Serotonin and suicidal behaviour. *Ann N Y Acad Sci* 1990;600:476–84.

19. Pandey GN, Dwivedi Y, Rizavi HS, *et al*. Higher expression of serotonin 5-HT$_{2A}$ receptors in the postmortem brains of teenage suicide victims. *Am J Psychiatry* 2002;1559:419–29.

20. Oquendo MA, Russo SA, Underwood MD, *et al*. Higher postmortem prefrontal 5-HT$_{2A}$ receptor binding correlates with lifetime aggression in suicide. *Biol Psychiatry* 2006;59:235–43.

21. Audenaert K, Van Laere K, Dumont F, *et al*. Decreased frontal serotonin 5-HT 2a receptor binding index in deliberate self-harm patients. *Eur J Nucl Med* 2001;28(2):175–82.

22. Van Heeringen K, Audenaert K, Van Laere K. Prefrontal 5-HT$_{2a}$ receptor binding index, hopelessness and personality characteristics in attempted suicide. *J Affect Disord* 2003;74:149–58.

23. Crowell SE, Beauchaine TP, McCauley E, *et al*. Psychological, autonomic and serotonergic correlates of parasuicide among adolescent girls. *Dev Psychopathol* 2005;17:1105–27.

24. Tyano S, Zalsman G, Ofek H, *et al*. Plasma serotonin levels and suicidal behaviour in adolescents. *Eur Neuropsychopharmacol* 2006;16:49–57.

25. Pfeffer CR, McBride PA, Anderson GM, *et al*. Peripheral serotonin measures in prepubertal psychiatric inpatients and normal children: associations with suicidal behaviour and its risk factors. *Biol Psychiatry* 1998;44:568–77.

26. Arango V, Underwood MD, Mann JJ. Fewer pigmented locus coeruleus neurons in suicide victims: preliminary results. *Biol Psychiatry* 1996;39:112–20.

27. Ordway GA, Widdowson PS, Streator Smith K, Halaris A. Agonist binding to α_2-adrenoceptors is elevated in the locus coeruleus from victims of suicide. *J Neurochem* 1994;63(2):617–24.

28. Agren H. Life at risk: markers of suicidality in depression. *Psychiatr Dev* 1983;1:87–103.

29. Van Heeringen K, Audenaert K, Van de Wiele L, Verstraete A. Cortisol in violent suicidal behaviour: association with personality and monoaminergic activity. *J Affect Disord* 2000;60:181–9.

30. Fawcett J, Busch KA, Jacobs D, *et al*. Suicide: a four-pathway clinical-biochemical model. *Ann N Y Acad Sci* 1997;836:288–301.

31. Coryell W, Schlesser M. The dexamethasone suppression test and suicide prediction. *Am J Psychiatry* 2001;158:748–53.

32. Pfeffer CR, Stokes P, Shinkdledecker R. Suicidal behaviour and hypothalamic-pituitary-adrenocortical axis indices in child psychiatric inpatients. *Biol Psychiatry* 1991;29:909–17.

33. Lopez LF, Vazquez DM, Chalmers DT, Watson SJ. Regulation of 5-HT receptors and the hypothalamic-pituitary-adrenal axis. Implications for the neurobiology of suicide. *Ann N Y Acad Sci* 1997;836:106–34.

34. Carballo JJ, Akamnonu CP, Oquendo MA. Neurobiology of suicidal behavior. An integration of biological and clinical findings. *Arch Suicide Res* 2008;12(2):93–110.

35. Pitchot W, Hansenne M, Ansseau M. Role of dopamine in non-depressed patients with a history of suicide attempts. *Eur Psychiatry* 2001;16:424–7.

36. Breese GR, Criswell HE, Mueller RA. Evidence that lack of brain dopamine during development can increase the susceptibility for aggression and self-injurious behavior by influencing the D_1-dopamine receptor function. *Prog Neuropsychopharmacol Biol Psychiatry* 1990;14:S65–80.

37. Schroeder SR, Oster-Granite ML, Berkson G, *et al.* Self-injurious behavior: gene-brain-behavior relationships. *Ment Retard Dev Disabil Res Rev* 2001;7:3–12.

38. Sivam SP. Dopamine, serotonin and tachykinin in self-injurious behaviour. *Life Sci* 1996;58(26):2367–75.

39. Herman BH. A possible role of proopiomelanocortin peptides in self-injurious behaviour. *Prog Neuropsychopharmacol Biol Psychiatry* 1990;14:S109–39.

40. Gross-Isseroff R, Dillon KA, Israeli M, Biegon A. Regionally selective increases in μ opiod receptor density in the brains of suicide victims. *Brain Res* 1990;530:312–6.

41. Pandey GN, Dwivedi Y, Rizavi HS, *et al.* Decreased catalytic activity and expression of protein kinase C isoenzymes in teenage suicide victims. *Arch Gen Psychiatry* 2004;61:685–93.

42. Young LT, Bezchlibnyk YB, Chen B, *et al.* Amygdala cyclic adenosine monophosphate response element binding protein phosphorylation in patients with mood disorders: effects of diagnosis, suicide, and drug treatment. *Biol Psychiatry* 2004;55:570–7.

43. Pacheco MA, Stockmeier C, Meltzer HY. Alterations in phosphoinositide signaling and G-protein levels in depressed suicide brain. *Brain Res* 1996;723:37–45.

44. Vinod KY, Hungund BL. Role of the endocannabinoid system in depression and suicide. *Trends Pharmacol Sci* 2006;27(10):539–45.

45. Deveci A, Aydemir O, Taskin O, *et al.* Serum BDNF levels in suicide attempters related to psychosocial stressors: a comparative study with depression. *Neuropsychobiology* 2007;56:93–7.

46. Karege F, Vaudan G, Schwald M, *et al.* Neurotrophin levels in postmortem brains of suicide victims and the effects of antemortem diagnosis and psychotropic drugs. *Brain Res Mol Brain Res* 2005;136:29–37.

47. Hibbeln JR, Umhau JC, George DT, *et al.* Plasma total cholesterol concentrations do not predict cerebrospinal fluid neurotransmitter metabolites: implications for the biophysical role of highly unsaturated fatty acids. *Am J Clin Nutr* 2000;71(Suppl 1):331S–8S.

48. Sublette ME, Hibbeln JR, Galfalvy H. Omega-3 polyunsaturated essential fatty acid status as a predictor of future suicide risk. *Am J Psychiatry* 2006;163(6):1100–2.

49. Brendel GR, Stern E, Silbersweig DA. Defining the neurocircuitry of borderline personality disorder: functional neuroimaging approaches. *Dev Psychopathol* 2005;17:1197–206.

50. Monkul ES, Hatch JP, Nicoletti MA, *et al.* Fronto-limbic brain structures in suicidal and non-suicidal female patients with major depressive disorder. *Mol Psychiatry* 2007;12:360–6.

CHAPTER 5

PSYCHOSOCIAL AND PSYCHIATRIC FACTORS RELATING TO ADOLESCENT SUICIDALITY AND SELF-HARM

Marinos Kyriakopoulos

Introduction

Suicidal behaviour has increasingly been recognised in the past three decades as a major public health concern. Suicide is one of the leading causes of death in adolescents and young adults worldwide[1-6] and takes a central part in the health policies of many countries including the UK.[7-9] The prevalence of self-harm has been extensively discussed in Chapter 2. Although completed suicide is relatively rare in adolescents,[5,6,10] it is still the second (after accidents) most common cause of death in this age group in most developed countries apart from USA, where it is also exceeded by homicide. However, self-harm[11-44] and suicidal thinking[13-16,19,25-26,29-33,45-46] are both common with the former being possibly on the rise.[11,47] In addition, self-harming is possibly on the rise.[11,47] Self-harm identification, detailed assessment and effective intervention in this age group, specifically taking into account their vulnerability, have been highlighted as public health imperatives.[48] These are dictated by the increased risk of suicide in young people engaging in self-harming behaviours[2,12,47] and the high co-occurrence of self-harm with mental health and social problems.[47]

Definitions

The difficulties in reaching a generally acceptable nomenclature in the field of suicidology[49-51] are discussed in detail in the first chapter of this book. The authors of the studies considered in this chapter use different definitions of self-harm. Some make a distinction between suicidal and non-suicidal self-harm and ideation and some do not. *Suicidal ideation* is generally defined as thoughts about killing oneself but in some studies might also include thoughts about non-suicidal self-harm. *Suicide attempt* refers to self-inflicted, potentially injurious behaviour with non-fatal outcome and evidence of explicit or inferred intent to die. *Non-suicidal self injury (NSSI) is defined as self-inflicted potentially injurious behaviour* where there is no evidence of explicit or inferred intent to die.[47,51] The term *self-harm* has been used in the UK to denote self-poisoning or self-injury irrespective of the apparent purpose of the specific act.[48] Self-harm in this context refers to acts directly intended to cause self-injury as an expression of personal distress rather than behaviours that are likely to cause harm (e.g. smoking, substance misuse) but are not adopted for this purpose.[48] *Suicidality* is the least clearly defined term and includes, in a broad sense, all thoughts and behaviours related to self-harm and in a narrower sense only those thoughts and behaviours relating to suicidal thoughts and behaviours. Finally, *suicide* is defined as a suicide attempt resulting in death.[51]

Psychosocial and psychiatric factors relating to adolescent suicidality and self-harm

Psychiatric disorders

Psychiatric disorders are strongly associated with a range of suicidal phenomena in adolescents.[52] About 60 per cent of under-16-year-olds and 90 per cent of older adolescents who complete suicide satisfy the diagnostic criteria for one or more psychiatric disorders.[53] Between 47 per cent and 74 per cent of adolescent suicides are attributable to mental disorder. Affective disorders (21–57 per cent) make the most substantial contribution.[54]

Mood disorders

Up to 60 per cent of adolescents who complete suicide have a depressive disorder.[55,56–63] There is an estimated 11- to 27-fold increase in the risk of completed suicide in this group compared with non-depressed adolescents.[2,55,59–61,63] Bipolar disorder in adolescence has not been consistently associated with completed suicide but some studies report this to be a risk factor.[58,61] Adolescents who attempt suicide show similar profiles to those who complete suicide with regard to depressive disorders,[64–67] but bipolar spectrum disorders in adolescence seem to be linked to a large increase in the risk of suicide attempts.[68,69] Major depressive disorder is probably the most common psychiatric diagnosis in adolescents who engage in NSSI, being diagnosable in up to 58 per cent of cases,[70–72] while other depressive disorders were also found to be prevalent.[70] However, a study directly comparing adolescent suicide attempters with those engaging in NSSI suggests that major depressive disorder may be more prevalent in the former group of adolescents.[73]

Anxiety and stress-related disorders

Anxiety disorders have been associated with suicidal ideation and attempts in adolescents and young adults.[64,65,74] However, the effects of anxiety disorders on suicidal behaviours as independent risk factors have been questioned,[55,64] while it has also been suggested that anxiety disorders need to be comorbid with depressive disorders in order to play a significant mediating role in these behaviours.[75,76] Post-traumatic stress disorder seems to be independently associated with suicidal ideation and attempts in adolescence even after controlling for depressive disorders.[77] Adolescents who engage in NSSI have similar rates of anxiety disorders to suicide attempters[70,73] but might have a higher prevalence of post-traumatic stress disorder (PTSD).[70]

Conduct disorders and substance misuse

Antisocial behaviour is linked with self-harm in adolescence. Completed suicide in conduct disorders is more likely if there is comorbid substance misuse.[55,61,78,63,79,80] Increased suicidal behaviour has also been associated with substance misuse[64,65,81–85] as well as with fire-setting in adolescents with conduct disorder.[86] A high percentage of adolescents who engage in NSSI also fulfil criteria for a conduct disorder,[38,70,73] although there is some evidence to suggest a lower rate of conduct disorder among the NSSI group than suicide attempters.[73]

Psychotic disorders

Suicidal ideation and attempts have been reported in children and adolescents with early-onset psychotic disorders.[87,88] The prevalence of ongoing suicide attempts and completed suicides seems to be increased in this group compared with the general population but suicides usually do not occur before adulthood.[89–91]

Other disorders

Suicidality and self-harm in adolescence have been associated with eating disorders,[55,64,81,92,93] attention deficit hyperactivity disorder (ADHD),[94,95] borderline personality disorder or traits[70,72,93,96] and other personality disorders.[66,96] Psychiatric comorbidity has been reported in adolescent suicide,[55,57,97] suicide attempts[64,65,75,76,81,83–85,98] and NSSI.[70,73]

No diagnosable disorder

Most studies of adolescent suicidal behaviour and NSSI identify a number of participants with no diagnosable mental disorder. In a US study[99] adolescent suicide in the absence of a diagnosable disorder was more likely to be the first suicidal act by an adolescent with a family history of affective illness, no past contact with services, increased rates of life stressors in the previous year and a higher likelihood of having a loaded gun at home. Compared with healthy adolescents this group showed a higher prevalence of mental illness in the family, past suicidal ideation or behaviour, discipline difficulties in the past 12 months and loaded firearm availability. Marttunen et al.[100] found less family disturbance, antisocial behaviour and contact with services in adolescents without a diagnosable disorder who committed suicide. Compared with adolescent suicide completers with a diagnosable disorder, this group was also found to have more discipline difficulties precipitating the suicide and to have communicated suicidal thoughts for the first time just before the act. Suicidal adolescents without diagnosable disorders from a large epidemiological sample[75] were found to have sub-threshold disruptive disorders. A proportion of these subjects also had impairing relationship difficulties, illicit drug use and alcohol use.

Physical illness

Suicidal behaviour has been reported in adolescents with epilepsy; depressive and conduct disorders probably are the mediating factors.[101,102] Suicide rates in adolescents with cancer are reported to be 1.8 times higher than rates in the general population.[103] Suicidal ideation may be increased in children and adolescents with insulin-dependent diabetes,[104,105] but this probably does not lead to higher than expected rates of suicide attempts[104,105] or suicide.[106] End-stage renal disease in young people does not seem to increase the likelihood of suicide.[107]

Interpersonal and psychological characteristics

Hopelessness

Of all the individual characteristics associated with suicidal behaviour and self-harm, hopelessness is probably the one that is most frequently reported. Adolescents attempting suicide were found to have elevated odds for hopelessness even after intercorrelations between hopelessness, neuroticism, introversion, low self-esteem, impulsiveness and an external locus of control were taken into account.[108] In addition, depressed adolescents who attempted suicide have been reported to experience significantly greater feelings of hopelessness than non-suicidal adolescents with depression.[109] Higher levels of hopelessness could differentiate adolescents who attempted suicide from those who only contemplated suicide, even though the groups had no difference in their scores on the Beck Depression Inventory.[110] Hopelessness was predictive of suicidal ideation in Hong Kong Chinese and Caucasian American adolescents in a study examining the associations between cognitive characteristics and depressive symptoms both cross-sectionally and longitudinally.[111] The association remained significant even after controlling for depressive symptoms; most notably hopelessness at baseline was predictive of suicidal ideation 6 months later, after demographics and baseline suicidal ideation were controlled for.[111] An independent predictive effect of hopelessness on suicide attempt repetition following an initial attempt during adolescence has also been identified in a longitudinal study involving mainly females.[112] High levels of hopelessness have also been associated with negative reinforcement leading to repetition of NSSI.[113] Hopelessness has been shown to have a direct effect as a mediator between social risk factors and suicidal behaviour in adolescents.[114] However, there are studies that reported these effects of hopelessness disappearing when severity of depression is controlled for. This was the case in the study by Hawton *et al.*,[115] where adolescents who repeatedly self-harmed scored higher for feelings of hopelessness than non-repeaters in univariate analysis and also in the study by Goldston *et al.*,[116] where hopelessness was predictive of suicide attempts post-hospitalisation in adolescents with a history of suicide attempts but not in those without. Feelings of hopelessness may also play a role in reduced help-seeking behaviour among those adolescents most in need of help.[117]

Impulsive aggression/anger

A higher degree of impulsive aggression, the individual characteristic of reacting aggressively when frustrated or challenged, has been associated with suicide[118] and suicidal behaviour[119] at a younger age, possibly also mediating the familial transmission of suicidal behaviour from parent to child.[119] Aggression may potentiate the effects of depression on suicide attempts in adolescence[120] and mediate suicidal ideation in adolescent eating disorders.[121] Anger and affect disregulation have been related to multiple suicide attempts after mood disorder was controlled for in a study comparing adolescents with a history of multiple suicide attempts with those who attempted suicide only once.[122] In addition, more residual anger was reported by adolescents with suicidal ideation than by those who attempted suicide during an acute suicidal episode.[110] This association between impulsive aggression or anger and suicidal behaviour in adolescents has not been found in all studies[123,124] or has been largely attenuated when severity of depression was controlled for.[115,125]

Impulsivity

Impulsivity has been associated with suicidality in adolescence but most studies have not found its effect to be independent of other variables, most notably depression.[108,115,124,126,127] Impulsivity may be related to death by suicide at an earlier age[118] and may be an important independent mediating factor in a subgroup of adolescents who engage in suicidal behaviours.[125]

Low self-esteem

Low self-esteem has been associated with suicidal behaviours in adolescence. In a sample of 487 adolescent inpatients low self-esteem was found to be, among other variables, an independent risk factor for suicidal behaviour.[126,128] Low self-esteem was a strong predictor for future suicide attempts in a representative community sample of more than 1500 older adolescents[129] and has also been associated with feelings of depression and suicidal behaviour in several studies.[108,115,125,127,130] These associations were generally attenuated after depression was controlled for. In addition, a study comparing three groups: depressed adolescents with a history of multiple suicide attempts; depressed adolescents who attempted suicide once and depressed adolescents who never attempted suicide, did not find differences in the levels of self-esteem.[109]

Neuroticism

Neuroticism is a personality trait associated with suicidal behaviour in adolescence and early adulthood. A longitudinal study of a birth cohort[108,131,130] showed neuroticism to be a risk factor for suicidality independent of other variables. Neuroticism was also related to suicidal ideation and was a predictor for the psychiatric readmission of adolescents hospitalised because of suicidal ideation.[132]

Problem-solving deficits

Adolescents who attempt suicide have been reported to have problem-solving deficits compared with non-suicidal psychiatric patients and healthy volunteers (for a review see ref. 133 and also refs 134 and 135). However, these deficits are associated with depression and hopelessness and the direction of causality is difficult to establish because of a lack of longitudinal studies examining these.

Addictive characteristics

Addictive characteristics of NSSI, most notably its negative reinforcement qualities and dependency elements, have been recognised.[113,136,137] In one study of hospitalised adolescents, dependency behaviours have been identified in almost all subjects engaging in NSSI, with the severity of the NSSI being associated with the urges and frequency of engaging in the behaviour.[138]

Other characteristics

Other personality characteristics reported to be risk factors for adolescent suicidality include perfectionism,[132] self-criticism,[132] external locus of control,[108] novelty seeking[131,130] and low self-image.[139,140] Self-isolation, not talking about one's own suicidal ideation and increased time with suicidal thoughts discriminated adolescents who attempted suicide from those with suicidal ideation alone.[110] Increased emotional reactivity[141] and thought suppression[142] have been associated with adolescent NSSI. Finally, certain survival and coping beliefs were identified as a protective factor in adolescent suicidality.[116]

Family factors

Family history

Family history of depression, suicidal behaviour, substance misuse and aggression have been associated with adolescent suicide and suicidal behaviours.[12,82,143–147] Suicidal behaviour was found to be increased in relatives of suicide probands compared with relatives of healthy control subjects after psychopathology was adjusted for.[144] The familial transmission of early-onset suicidal behaviour seems to be independent of the transmission of psychiatric disorder[147,148] whereas familial loading for suicidality is associated with earlier onset of suicidal behaviours.[146,149,150] Adoption and twin studies support the involvement of genetic factors in familial transmission of suicidal behaviour, with estimated heritability ranging between 38 per cent and 55 per cent.[147]

Family structure and relationships

Adolescents engaging in suicidal behaviour, including suicide, are more likely to come from non-intact families and disadvantaged or dysfunctional family environments.[82,98,130,145,146,151,152] These associations may be, at least partly, explained by parental mental illness leading to more adversity within the family. However, several factors including poor parent–child communication,[145,152] having a father exerting control without affection,[153] poor family environment and low parental monitoring,[146] living away from parents[33] and family socioeconomic adversity[130] emerged as also having independent negative effects on adolescent suicidality. In addition, adoption has been reported to be a risk factor for suicide attempts during adolescence, even after adjusting for depression and aggression.[139] Parental expressed emotions, and most specifically criticism, have also been identified as being strongly associated with thoughts and behaviours about self-harm in adolescents as a whole but also separately with suicidal thoughts, behaviours and NSSI.[154] These associations were not explained by the presence of mental disorders.

Parental bereavement

Parental bereavement, especially before the age of 12 years, has been associated with depression and suicidal behaviour in adolescents.[155] It has been suggested that adolescent suicide in parental bereavement is more likely in cases of paternal death by suicide and maternal death by any cause (but more so when by suicide).[151] In addition, the offspring of parents who died of suicide have more severe psychopathology than the offspring of parents who died of cancer[156] or other causes.[157] However, most studies do not support this link between parental death by suicide, as opposed to other causes, and increased suicidal behaviour in the offspring,[157–159] while, as already mentioned, there are other possible explanations for the familial transmission of suicidal behaviour.[147]

Sexual orientation

Suicide was not associated with homosexuality in one psychological autopsy study looking at 120 out of 170 consecutive suicides in young people under the age of 20 years and 147 community-matched healthy control subjects in the Greater New York City area,[160] but only three suicide completers and no control subjects met study criteria for homosexuality. However, several studies have identified a strong link between non-heterosexual orientation and mental health problems, including suicidality in adolescence.[161–166] Suicidal thoughts and attempts in this group seem to be associated to an extent with stressors around the young people's sexual orientation, such as becoming aware of same-sex feelings[167] and admission of sexual orientation to others including parents.[167,168] Identified risk factors particularly relevant to gay, lesbian and bisexual suicidality include early gender-atypical behaviour, early openness about sexual orientation, parental pressure discouraging gender-atypical behaviour,[168] loss of friends and victimisation after disclosure of sexual orientation.[169] It has also been suggested that gender non-conformity may be a risk factor associated more strongly with male adolescent suicidality.[170,171] It must be noted that 84.6 per cent of male and 71.7 per cent of female young people with non-heterosexual orientation report no suicidal thoughts or behaviours.[2]

Maltreatment

The link between child and adolescent maltreatment mainly in the form of sexual, but also physical, abuse and suicidality is a very consistent finding in the literature.[16,131,130,163,170–177] Although it has been suggested that the effects of maltreatment are mediated by other factors, including mental health, interpersonal or social problems,[130,171] several studies report an independent effect of abuse on self-harm in adolescence and young adulthood[16,131,163,170–174,176,177] while some studies also found a dose–response relationship between severity of maltreatment and suicidality.[172,174] The exploration of the complex relationship between child sexual abuse and the familial transmission of suicidal behaviour has shown that child sexual abuse is a risk factor for suicidality both to the person suffering it and to their offspring.[178] This may be partly explained by the familial transmission of child sexual abuse, possibly through factors related to interactions within the family.[178] Protective factors that reduce the risk of self-harm following child sexual abuse include family connectedness, a caring relationship with an adult, a parent or a teacher, good peer relationships, school safety and school achievement.[131,163,171] Finally, physical neglect, emotional abuse and sexual abuse are associated with NSSI in adolescence; self-criticism seems to play a mediating role.[179]

Social factors

Social support and peer relationships

Several factors associated with social support systems other than the family have been identified as very relevant in adolescent suicidal behaviour, even after current psychopathology was taken into account. School problems, school violence and bullying have been highlighted as independent risk factors in many studies.[20,140,145,180–182] Interestingly, both young people who bully others and those who are victims of bullying are at increased risk for depression, suicidal thoughts and behaviours.[181,183,184] Of the different types of victimisation, being belittled about looks and speech in females, being belittled about religion and race in males, being physically bullied, being the subject of rumours and 'mean lies', being the subject of sexual jokes, comments and gestures, and cyber victimisation were significantly associated with adolescent suicidality.[184] A higher risk for suicidal behaviour was associated with an increasing number of the types of victimisation in a dose–response manner.[184] Individual psychopathology has been linked to bullying, both in and out of school, with those adolescents who are both bullies and victims being the most affected.[181] School connectedness[20,185] and having friends[180] have been identified as protective factors for suicide attempts in adolescence.

Exposure to suicidal behaviour

Exposure to a suicide attempt by a friend or family member has been associated with an increased risk of self-harm in adolescents.[33,127,155] However, exposure to the suicide of a friend does not seem to influence the risk of suicide attempts in the peer group, but it may have longer-term effects, increasing the risk of depression, anxiety and PTSD.[186] The increased incidence of suicidal behaviours in friends of adolescents attempting suicide may be explained by imitation and influence between friends but also by a possible tendency of young people with mental health problems to form friendships between themselves.[187] Contagion of suicidal behaviour has also been supported by studies of suicide clusters and the effect of the media on suicidality. Significant temporal and spatial clustering of suicides and suicide attempts has been reported in adolescents and young adults.[188–191] The degree of media coverage of suicide stories seems to be related to suicide increases, especially among adolescents (for a review see ref. 192). The form and content of the coverage are important factors affecting the risk of imitation. Front-page reporting, large headlines, many pictures and the repetition of the story over many days have been considered to be imitation risk factors.[192] Stories about group suicides and suicide following homicide do not seem to have a significant imitation effect, while greater potential for identification with the suicide victim, e.g. via reporting of the victim's marital problems, or a romanticising of the suicide, are more likely to lead to imitation.[192] This association between media coverage of suicide and suicide incidence in the population has been reported in many countries.[192]

Availability of means

The restriction on the availability of lethal means has been pursued on the assumption that suicidality is transient and related to impulsivity.[193] Individuals who attempt suicide may be ambivalent and not have an enduring wish to die; therefore, their death can be the accidental outcome of an impulsive suicide attempt using a lethal method.[193] Public health measures such as legislation to limit the size of analgesic packs in the UK have led to substantial reductions in non-fatal overdoses.[193,194] This may be particularly important in the prevention of fatal overdoses in adolescence, since paracetamol is the most common method of self-poisoning in younger ages.[11,37] In the USA, restrictions on firearms, a significant risk factor for suicide in young people,[97,60,195] have resulted in reported reductions of gun-related suicides and the overall suicide rates in most studies.[2] Similar reductions in gun-related suicides after the introduction of increased firearm restrictions have been reported in other countries.[196,197]

Religiosity

Several studies have suggested that religiosity and frequent worship attendance both have a protective role in relation to suicidal behaviours in adolescents and young adults.[20,163,198-201] This effect may not be independent of cultural and relational aspects in religious individuals and groups and can possibly be explained by indirect suicide prevention through the prohibition of substance abuse, better social support and integration, and protective beliefs about the sacredness and meaning of life.

Conclusions

Adolescent suicide and self-harm are the result of complex interactions between interpersonal, social and psychiatric factors. Several lines of research in the last 30 years have significantly increased our insight into their mechanisms and outcomes. A better understanding of their pathways is the first step towards comprehensive evaluation, effective intervention and prevention of suicidal and self-harming behaviours in young people.

References

1. Carr A, editor. *Prevention: what works with children and adolescents? A critical review of psychological prevention programmes for children, adolescents and their families.* Hove, UK: Brunner-Routledge; 2002.
2. Gould MS, Greenberg T, Velting DM, Shaffer D. Youth suicide risk and preventive interventions: a review of the past 10 years. *J Am Acad Child Adolesc Psychiatry* 2003;**42**(4):386–405.
3. Jenkins R. Addressing suicide as a public-health problem. *Lancet* 20029;**359**(9309):813–4.
4. Kochanek KD, Murphy SL, Anderson RN, Scott C. *Natl Vital Stat Rep* 2004;**53**(5):1–115.
5. Phillips MR, Li X, Zhang Y. Suicide rates in China, 1995–99. *Lancet* 2002; **359**(9309): 835–40.
6. World Health Organization, 2003 [accessed 12 December 2008] Available from: http://www.who.int/mental_health/prevention/suicide.
7. DH. *National suicide prevention strategy for England.* London, UK: Department of Health; 2002.
8. DH. *Choosing health.* London, UK: Department of Health; 2004.
9. DH. *The national service framework for mental health. Modern standards and service models for mental health.* London, UK: Department of Health; 1999.
10. Windfuhr K, While D, Hunt I, *et al.* National Confidential Inquiry into Suicide and Homicide by People with Mental Illness. Suicide in juveniles and adolescents in the United Kingdom. *J Child Psychol Psychiatry.* 2008;**49**(11):1155–65.
11. Hawton K, Harriss L. Deliberate self-harm by under-15-year-olds: characteristics, trends and outcome. *J Child Psychol Psychiatry* 2008;**49**(4):441–8.

12. Bridge JA, Goldstein TR, Brent DA. Adolescent suicide and suicidal behavior. *J Child Psychol Psychiatry* 2006;**47**(3,4):372–94.

13. Madge N, Hewitt A, Hawton K, *et al*. Deliberate self-harm within an international community sample of young people: comparative findings from the Child & Adolescent Self-harm in Europe (CASE) Study. *J Child Psychol Psychiatry* 2008;**49**(6):667–77.

14. Alaimo K, Olson CM, Frongillo EA. Family food insufficiency, but not low family income, is positively associated with dysthymia and suicide symptoms in adolescents. *J Nutr* 2002;**132**(4):719–25.

15. Eisenberg ME, Neumark-Sztainer D, Story M. Associations of weight-based teasing and emotional well-being among adolescents. *Arch Pediatr Adolesc Med* 2003;**157**(8):733–8

16. Waldrop AE, Hanson RF, Resnick HS, *et al*. Risk factors for suicidal behavior among a national sample of adolescents: implications for prevention. *J Trauma Stress* 2007;**20**(5):869–79.

17. Olsson GI, von Knorring AL. Adolescent depression: prevalence in Swedish high-school students. *Acta Psychiatr Scand* 1999;**99**(5):324–31.

18. Elklit A. Victimization and PTSD in a Danish national youth probability sample. *J Am Acad Child Adolesc Psychiatry* 2002;**41**(2):174–81.

19. Gmitrowicz A, Szymczak W, Kropiwnicki P, Rabe-Jablonska J. Gender influence in suicidal behaviour of Polish adolescents. *Eur Child Adolesc Psychiatry* 2003;**12**(5):205–13.

20. Blum RW, Halcon L, Beuhring T, Pate E, Campell-Forrester S, Venema A. Adolescent health in the Caribbean: risk and protective factors. *Am J Public Health* 2003;**93**(3):456–60.

21. Toros F, Bilgin NG, Sasmaz T, *et al*. Suicide attempts and risk factors among children and adolescents. *Yonsei Med J* 2004;**45**(3):367–74.

22. Zemaitiene N, Zaborskis A. Suicidal tendencies and attitude towards freedom to choose suicide among Lithuanian schoolchildren: results from three cross-sectional studies in 1994, 1998, and 2002. *BMC Public Health* 2005;**5**:83.

23. Young R, Sweeting H, West P. Prevalence of deliberate self-harm and attempted suicide within contemporary Goth youth subculture: longitudinal cohort study. *BMJ* 2006;**332**(7549):1058–61.

24. Silviken A, Kvernmo S. Suicide attempts among indigenous Sami adolescents and majority peers in Arctic Norway: prevalence and associated risk factors. *J Adolesc* 2007;**30**(4): 613–26.

25. Sidhartha T, Jena S. Suicidal behaviors in adolescents. *Indian J Pediatr* 2006;**73**(9):783–8.

26. Centers for Disease Control and Prevention. National Youth Risk Behavior Survey: 1991–2005: trends in the prevalence of suicide ideation and attempts. Atlanta (GA): Centers for Disease Control and Prevention, 2007 [accessed 20 December 2008] Available from: http://www.cdc.gov/HealthyYouth/yrbs/pdf/trends/2005_YRBS_Suicide_Attempts.pdf.

27. Tousignant M, Habimana E, Biron C, *et al*. The Quebec Adolescent Refugee Project: psychopathology and family variables in a sample from 35 nations. *J Am Acad Child Adolesc Psychiatry* 1999;**38**(11):1426–32.

28. Miauton L, Narring F, Michaud PA. Chronic illness, life style and emotional health in adolescence: results of a cross-sectional survey on the health of 15–20-year-olds in Switzerland. *Eur J Pediatr* 2003;**162**(10):682–9.

29. Yip PS, Liu KY, Lam TH, *et al*. Suicidality among high school students in Hong Kong, SAR. *Suicide Life Threat Behav* 2004;**34**(3):284–97.

30. Rodriguez AH, Caldera T, Kullgren G, Renberg ES. Suicidal expressions among young people in Nicaragua: a community-based study. *Soc Psychiatry Psychiatr Epidemiol* 2006;**41**(9):692–7.

31. Rudatsikira E, Muula AS, Siziya S. Prevalence and associated factors of suicidal ideation among school-going adolescents in Guyana: results from a cross sectional study. *Clin Pract Epidemol Ment Health* 2007;3:13.

32. O'Donnell L, O'Donnell C, Wardlaw DM, Stueve A. Risk and resiliency factors influencing suicidality among urban African American and Latino youth. *Am J Community Psychol* 2004;33(1,2):37–49.

33. Rey Gex C, Narring F, Ferron C, Michaud PA. Suicide attempts among adolescents in Switzerland: prevalence, associated factors and comorbidity. *Acta Psychiatr Scand* 1998;98(1):28–33.

34. Nock MK, Borges G, Bromet EJ, *et al*. Suicide and suicidal behavior. *Epidemiol Rev* 2008;30:133–54.

35. Eaton DK, Kann L, Kinchen S, *et al*. Centers for Disease Control and Prevention (CDC). Youth risk behavior surveillance – United States, 2007. *MMWR Surveill Summ* 2008;57(4):1–131.

36. Hultén A, Jiang GX, Wasserman D, *et al*. Repetition of attempted suicide among teenagers in Europe: frequency, timing and risk factors. *Eur Child Adolesc Psychiatry* 2001;10(3):161–9.

37. Hawton K, Harriss L. Deliberate self-harm in young people: characteristics and subsequent mortality in a 20-year cohort of patients presenting to hospital. *J Clin Psychiatry* 2007;68(10):1574–83.

38. Laye-Gindhu A, Schonert-Reichl KA. Nonsuicidal self-harm among community adolescents: Understanding the 'whats' and 'whys' of self-harm. *J Youth Adolesc* 2005;34(5):447–57.

39. Muehlenkamp JJ, Gutierrez PM. An investigation of differences between self-injurious behavior and suicide attempts in a sample of adolescents. *Suicide Life Threat Behav* 2004;34(1):12–23.

40. Muehlenkamp JJ, Gutierrez PM. Risk for suicide attempts among adolescents who engage in non-suicidal self-injury. *Arch Suicide Res* 2007;11(1):69–82.

41. Ross S, Heath N. Two models of adolescent self-mutilation. *Suicide Life Threat Behav* 2003;33(3):277–87.

42. Zoroglu SS, Tuzun U, Sar V, *et al*. Suicide attempt and self-mutilation among Turkish high school students in relation with abuse, neglect, and dissociation. *Psychiatry Clin Neurosci* 2003;57(1):119–26.

43. Whitlock J, Eckenrode J, Silverman D. Self-injurious behaviors in a college population. *Pediatrics* 2006;117(6):1939–48.

44. Lloyd-Richardson E, Perrine N, Dierker L, Kelley ML. Characteristics and functions of non-suicidal self-injury in a community sample of adolescents. *Psychol Med* 2007;37(8):1183–92.

45. Dervic K, Akkaya-Kalayci T, Kapusta ND, *et al*. Suicidal ideation among Viennese high school students. *Wien Klin Wochenschr* 2007;119(5–6):174–80.

46. Kaltiala-Heino R, Rimpela M, Marttunen M, *et al*. Bullying, depression, and suicidal ideation in Finnish adolescents: school survey. *BMJ* 1999;319(7206):348–51.

47. Jacobson CM, Gould M. The epidemiology and phenomenology of non-suicidal self-injurious behavior among adolescents: a critical review of the literature. *Arch Suicide Res* 2007;11(2):129–47.

48. NICE. Self-harm: the short-term physical and psychological management and secondary prevention of self-harm in primary and secondary care. London, UK: National Institute of Clinical Excellence; 2004.

49. Silverman MM. The language of suicidology. *Suicide Life Threat Behav* 2006;36(5): 519–32.

50. Silverman MM, Berman AL, Sanddal ND, O'carroll PW, Joiner TE. Rebuilding the tower of Babel: a revised nomenclature for the study of suicide and suicidal behaviors. Part 2: suicide-related ideations, communications, and behaviors. *Suicide Life Threat Behav* 2007;37(3):264–77.

51. Silverman MM, Berman AL, Sanddal ND, *et al.* Rebuilding the tower of Babel: a revised nomenclature for the study of suicide and suicidal behaviors. Part 1: background, rationale, and methodology. *Suicide Life Threat Behav* 2007;37(3):248–63.

52. Evans E, Hawton K, Rodham K, *et al.* Factors associated with suicidal phenomena in adolescents: a systematic review of population-based studies. *Clin Psychol Rev* 2004;24(8):957–79.

53. Brent DA, Baugher M, Bridge J, *et al.* Age- and sex-related risk factors for adolescent suicide. *J Am Acad Child Adolesc Psychiatry* 1999;38(12):1497–505.

54. Cavanagh JT, Carson AJ, Sharpe M, *et al.* Psychological autopsy studies of suicide: a systematic review.[Erratum appears in *Psychol Med* 2003;33(5):947.] *Psychol Med* 2003;33(3):395–405.

55. Shaffer D, Gould MS, Fisher P, *et al.* Psychiatric diagnosis in child and adolescent suicide. *Arch Gen Psychiatry* 1996;53(4):339–48

56. Beautrais AL. Child and young adolescent suicide in New Zealand. *Aust N Z J Psychiatry* 2001;35(5):647–53.

57. Fleischmann A, Bertolote JM, Belfer M, Beautrais A. Completed suicide and psychiatric diagnoses in young people: a critical examination of the evidence. *Am J Orthopsychiatry* 2005;75(4):676–83.

58. Marttunen MJ, Aro HM, Henriksson MM, Lonnqvist JK. Mental disorders in adolescent suicide. DSM-III-R axes I and II diagnoses in suicides among 13- to 19-year-olds in Finland.. *Arch Gen Psychiatry* 1991;48(9):834–9.

59. Shafii M, Steltz-Lenarsky J, Derrick AM, *et al.* Comorbidity of mental disorders in the post-mortem diagnosis of completed suicide in children and adolescents. *J Affect Disord* 1988;15(3):227–33.

60. Brent DA, Perper JA, Goldstein CE, *et al.* Risk factors for adolescent suicide: a comparison of adolescent suicide victims with suicidal inpatients. *Arch Gen Psychiatry* 1988;45(6):581–8.

61. Brent DA, Perper JA, Moritz G, *et al.* Psychiatric risk factors for adolescent suicide: a case-control study. *J Am Acad Child Adolesc Psychiatry* 1993;32(3):521–9.

62. Apter A, Bleich A, King RA, *et al.* Death without warning? A clinical postmortem study of suicide in 43 Israeli adolescent males. *Arch Gen Psychiatry* 1993;50(2):138–42.

63. Groholt B, Ekeberg O, Wichstrom L, Haldorsen T. Suicide among children and younger and older adolescents in Norway: a comparative study. *J Am Acad Child Adolesc Psychiatry* 1998;37(5):473–81.

64. Beautrais AL, Joyce PR, Mulder RT. Risk factors for serious suicide attempts among youths aged 13 through 24 years. *J Am Acad Child Adolesc Psychiatry* 1996;35(9): 1174–82.

65. Gould MS, King R, Greenwald S, *et al.* Psychopathology associated with suicidal ideation and attempts among children and adolescents. *J Am Acad Child Adolesc Psychiatry* 1998;37(9):915–23.

66. Portzky G, Audenaert K, van Heeringen K. Psychosocial and psychiatric factors associated

with adolescent suicide: a case-control psychological autopsy study. *J Adolesc* 2008 Nov 20. [Epub ahead of print] doi:10.1016/j.adolescence.2008.10.007

67. Fordwood SR, Asarnow JR, Huizar DP, Reise SP. Suicide attempts among depressed adolescents in primary care. *J Clin Child Adolesc Psychol* 2007;36(3):392–404.

68. Goldstein TR, Birmaher B, Axelson D, *et al*. History of suicide attempts in pediatric bipolar disorder: factors associated with increased risk. *Bipolar Disord* 2005;7(6):525–35.

69. Lewinsohn PM, Klein DN, Seeley JR. Bipolar disorders in a community sample of older adolescents: prevalence, phenomenology, comorbidity, and course. *J Am Acad Child Adolesc Psychiatry* 1995;34(4):454–63.

70. Jacobson CM, Muehlenkamp JJ, Miller AL, Turner JB. Psychiatric impairment among adolescents engaging in different types of deliberate self-harm. *J Clin Child Adolesc Psychol* 2008;37(2):363–75.

71. Kumar G, Pepe D, Steer RA. Adolescent psychiatric inpatients' self-reported reasons for cutting themselves. *J Nerv Ment Dis* 2004;192(12):830–6.

72. Nock MK, Joiner TE, Jr, Gordon KH, *et al*. Non-suicidal self-injury among adolescents: diagnostic correlates and relation to suicide attempts. *Psychiatry Res* 2006 Sep 30;144(1):65–72.

73. Nock MK, Kessler RC. Prevalence of and risk factors for suicide attempts versus suicide gestures: analysis of the National Comorbidity Survey. *J Abnorm Psychol* 2006;115(3):616–23.

74. Boden JM, Fergusson DM, Horwood LJ. Anxiety disorders and suicidal behaviours in adolescence and young adulthood: findings from a longitudinal study. *Psychol Med* 2007;37(3):431–40.

75. Foley DL, Goldston DB, Costello EJ, Angold A. Proximal psychiatric risk factors for suicidality in youth: the Great Smoky Mountains Study. *Arch Gen Psychiatry* 2006;63(9):1017–24.

76. Tuisku V, Pelkonen M, Karlsson L, *et al*. Suicidal ideation, deliberate self-harm behaviour and suicide attempts among adolescent outpatients with depressive mood disorders and comorbid axis I disorders. *Eur Child Adolesc Psychiatry* 2006;15(4):199–206.

77. Mazza JJ. The relationship between posttraumatic stress symptomatology and suicidal behavior in school-based adolescents. *Suicide Life Threat Behav* 2000;30(2):91–103.

78. de Chateau P. Mortality and aggressiveness in a 30-year follow-up study in child guidance clinics in Stockholm. *Acta Psychiatr Scand* 1990;81(5):472–6.

79. Kuperman S, Black DW, Burns TL. Excess suicide among formerly hospitalized child psychiatry patients. *J Clin Psychiatry* 1988;49(3):88–93.

80. Renaud J, Brent DA, Birmaher B, *et al*. Suicide in adolescents with disruptive disorders. *J Am Acad Child Adolesc Psychiatry* 1999;38(7):846–51.

81. Andrews JA, Lewinsohn PM. Suicidal attempts among older adolescents: Prevalence and co-occurrence with psychiatric disorders. *J Am Acad Child Adolesc Psychiatry* 1992;31(4):655–62.

82. Fergusson DM, Lynskey MT. Suicide attempts and suicidal ideation in a birth cohort of 16-year-old New Zealanders. *J Am Acad Child Adolesc Psychiatry* 1995;34(10):1308–17.

83. Haavisto A, Sourander A, Ellilä H, *et al*. Suicidal ideation and suicide attempts among child and adolescent psychiatric inpatients in Finland. *J Affect Disord* 2003;76(1–3):211–21.

84. Ilomäki E, Räsänen P, Viilo K, Hakko H: STUDY-70 Workgroup. Suicidal behavior among adolescents with conduct disorder – the role of alcohol dependence. *Psychiatry Res* 2007;150(3):305–11.

85. Garrison CZ, McKeown RE, Valois RF, Vincent ML. Aggression, substance use, and suicidal behaviors in high school students. *Am J Public Health* 1993;83(2):179–84.

86. Martin G, Bergen HA, Richardson AS, *et al.* Correlates of firesetting in a community sample of young adolescents. *Aust N Z J Psychiatry* 2004;38(3):148–54.

87. Asarnow JR, Tompson MC, Goldstein MJ. Childhood-onset schizophrenia: a followup study. *Schizophr Bull* 1994;20(4):599–617.

88. Schwartz-Stav O, Apter A, Zalsman G. Depression, suicidal behavior and insight in adolescents with schizophrenia. *Eur Child Adolesc Psychiatry* 2006;15(6):352–9

89. Jarbin H, Von Knorring AL. Suicide and suicide attempts in adolescent-onset psychotic disorders. *Nord J Psychiatry* 2004;58(2):115–23.

90. Kotila L, Lönnqvist J. Suicide and violent death among adolescent suicide attempters. *Acta Psychiatr Scand* 1989;79(5):453–9.

91. Remschmidt H, Martin M, Fleischhaker C, *et al.* Forty-two-years later: the outcome of childhood-onset schizophrenia. *J Neural Transm* 2007;114(4):505–12.

92. Fischer S, le Grange D. Comorbidity and high-risk behaviors in treatment-seeking adolescents with bulimia nervosa. *Int J Eat Disord* 2007;40(8):751–3

93. Ohmann S, Schuch B, Konig M, *et al.* Self-injurious behavior in adolescent girls. Association with psychopathology and neuropsychological functions. *Psychopathology* 2008;41(4):226–35.

94. Goodman G, Gerstadt C, Pfeffer CR, *et al.* ADHD and aggression as correlates of suicidal behavior in assaultive prepubertal psychiatric inpatients. *Suicide Life Threat Behav* 2008;38(1):46–59.

95. James A, Lai FH, Dahl C. Attention deficit hyperactivity disorder and suicide: a review of possible associations. *Acta Psychiatr Scand* 2004;110(6):408–15.

96. Brent DA, Johnson BA, Perper J, *et al.* Personality disorder, personality traits, impulsive violence, and completed suicide in adolescents. *J Am Acad Child Adolesc Psychiatry* 1994;33(8):1080–6.

97. Brent DA, Baugher M, Bridge J, *et al.* Age- and sex-related risk factors for adolescent suicide. *J Am Acad Child Adolesc Psychiatry* 1999;38(12):1497–505.

98. Fergusson DM, Lynskey MT. Childhood circumstances, adolescent adjustment, and suicide attempts in a New Zealand birth cohort. *J Am Acad Child Adolesc Psychiatry* 1995;34(5):612–22.

99. Brent DA, Perper J, Moritz G, *et al.* Suicide in adolescents with no apparent psychopathology. *J Am Acad Child Adolesc Psychiatry* 1993;32(3):494–500.

100. Marttunen MJ, Henriksson MM, Isometsä ET, *et al.* Completed suicide among adolescents with no diagnosable psychiatric disorder. *Adolescence* 1998 Fall;33(131):669–81.

101. Baker GA. Depression and suicide in adolescents with epilepsy. *Neurology* 2006;66(6 Suppl 3):S5–12.

102. Caplan R, Siddarth P, Gurbani S, Hanson R, Sankar R, Shields WD. Depression and anxiety disorders in pediatric epilepsy. *Epilepsia* 2005;46(5):720–30.

103. Misono S, Weiss NS, Fann JR, *et al.* Incidence of suicide in persons with cancer. *J Clin Oncol* 2008;26(29):4731–8.

104. Goldston DB, Kelley AE, Reboussin DM, *et al.* Suicidal ideation and behavior and noncompliance with the medical regimen among diabetic adolescents. *J Am Acad Child Adolesc Psychiatry* 1997;36(11):1528–36.

105. Goldston DB, Kovacs M, Ho VY, *et al.* Suicidal ideation and suicide attempts among youth with insulin-dependent diabetes mellitus. *J Am Acad Child Adolesc Psychiatry* 1994;33(2):240–6.

106. Dahlquist G, Källén B. Mortality in childhood-onset type 1 diabetes: a population-based study. *Diabetes Care* 2005;**28**(10):2384–7.

107. Kurella M, Kimmel PL, Young BS, Chertow GM. Suicide in the United States end-stage renal disease program. *J Am Soc Nephrol* 2005;**16**(3):774–81.

108. Beautrais AL, Joyce PR, Mulder RT. Personality traits and cognitive styles as risk factors for serious suicide attempts among young people. *Suicide Life Threat Behav* 1999;**29**(1):37–47.

109. Dori GA, Overholser JC. Depression, hopelessness, and self-esteem: accounting for suicidality in adolescent psychiatric inpatients. *Suicide Life Threat Behav* 1999;**29**(4): 309–18.

110. Negron R, Piacentini J, Graae F, *et al.* Microanalysis of adolescent suicide attempters and ideators during the acute suicidal episode. *J Am Acad Child Adolesc Psychiatry* 1997;**36**(11):1512–9.

111. Stewart SM, Kennard BD, Lee PW, *et al.* Hopelessness and suicidal ideation among adolescents in two cultures. *J Child Psychol Psychiatry* 2005;**46**(4):364–72.

112. Groholt B, Ekeberg Ø, Haldorsen T. Adolescent suicide attempters: what predicts future suicidal acts? *Suicide Life Threat Behav* 2006;**36**(6):638–50.

113. Nock MK, Prinstein MJ. Contextual features and behavioral functions of self-mutilation among adolescents. *J Abnorm Psychol* 2005;**114**(1):140–6.

114. Thompson EA, Mazza JJ, Herting JR, *et al.* The mediating roles of anxiety, depression, and hopelessness on adolescent suicidal behaviors. *Suicide Life Threat Behav* 2005;**35**(1):14–34.

115. Hawton K, Kingsbury S, Steinhardt K, *et al.* Repetition of deliberate self-harm by adolescents: the role of psychological factors. *J Adolesc* 1999;**22**(3):369–78.

116. Goldston DB, Daniel SS, Reboussin BA, *et al.* Cognitive risk factors and suicide attempts among formerly hospitalized adolescents: a prospective naturalistic study. *J Am Acad Child Adolesc Psychiatry* 2001;**40**(1):91–9.

117. Gould MS, Greenberg T, Munfakh JL, *et al.* Teenagers' attitudes about seeking help from telephone crisis services (hotlines). *Suicide Life Threat Behav* 2006;**36**(6):601–13.

118. McGirr A, Renaud J, Bureau A, *et al.* Impulsive-aggressive behaviours and completed suicide across the life cycle: a predisposition for younger age of suicide. *Psychol Med* 2008;**38**(3):407–17.

119. Melhem NM, Brent DA, Ziegler M, *et al.* Familial pathways to early-onset suicidal behavior: familial and individual antecedents of suicidal behavior. *Am J Psychiatry* 2007;**164**(9):1364–70.

120. Kerr DC, Washburn JJ, Feingold A, *et al.* Sequelae of aggression in acutely suicidal adolescents. *J Abnorm Child Psychol* 2007;**35**(5):817–30.

121. Miotto P, Preti A. Eating disorders and suicide ideation: the mediating role of depression and aggressiveness. *Compr Psychiatry* 2007;**48**(3):218–24.

122. Esposito C, Spirito A, Boergers J, Donaldson D. Affective, behavioral, and cognitive functioning in adolescents with multiple suicide attempts. *Suicide Life Threat Behav* 2003;**33**(4):389–99.

123. Brent DA, Johnson B, Bartle S, *et al.* Personality disorder, tendency to impulsive violence, and suicidal behavior in adolescents. *J Am Acad Child Adolesc Psychiatry* 1993;**32**(1):69–75.

124. Renaud J, Berlim MT, McGirr A, *et al.* Current psychiatric morbidity, aggression/impulsivity, and personality dimensions in child and adolescent suicide: a case-control study. *J Affect Disord* 2008;**105**(1–3):221–8.

125. Kingsbury S, Hawton K, Steinhardt K, James A. Do adolescents who take overdoses have specific psychological characteristics? A comparative study with psychiatric and community controls. *J Am Acad Child Adolesc Psychiatry* 1999;38(9):1125–31.

126. Becker DF, Grilo CM. Prediction of suicidality and violence in hospitalized adolescents: comparisons by sex. *Can J Psychiatry* 2007;52(9):572–80.

127. Hawton K, Rodham K, Evans E, Weatherall R. Deliberate self-harm in adolescents: self report survey in schools in England. *BMJ* 2002 Nov 23;325(7374):1207–11.

128. Overholser JC, Adams DM, Lehnert KL, Brinkman DC. Self-esteem deficits and suicidal tendencies among adolescents. *J Am Acad Child Adolesc Psychiatry* 1995;34(7):919–28.

129. Lewinsohn PM, Rohde P, Seeley JR. Psychosocial risk factors for future adolescent suicide attempts. *J Consult Clin Psychol* 1994;62(2):297–305.

130. Fergusson DM, Woodward LJ, Horwood LJ. Risk factors and life processes associated with the onset of suicidal behaviour during adolescence and early adulthood. *Psychol Med* 2000;30(1):23–39.

131. Fergusson DM, Beautrais AL, Horwood LJ. Vulnerability and resiliency to suicidal behaviours in young people. *Psychol Med* 2003;33(1):61–73.

132. Enns MW, Cox BJ, Inayatulla M. Personality predictors of outcome for adolescents hospitalized for suicidal ideation. *J Am Acad Child Adolesc Psychiatry* 2003;42(6):720–7.

133. Speckens AE, Hawton K. Social problem solving in adolescents with suicidal behavior: a systematic review. *Suicide Life Threat Behav* 2005;35(4):365–87.

134. Arie M, Apter A, Orbach I, *et al.* Autobiographical memory, interpersonal problem solving, and suicidal behavior in adolescent inpatients. *Compr Psychiatry* 2008;49(1):22–9.

135. Crane C, Barnhofer T, Williams JM. Reflection, brooding, and suicidality: a preliminary study of different types of rumination in individuals with a history of major depression. *Br J Clin Psychol* 2007;46(Pt 4):497–504.

136. Faye P. Addictive characteristics of the behavior of self-mutilation. *J Psychosoc Nurs Ment Health Serv* 1995;33(6):36–9.

137. Karwautz A, Resch F, Wöber-Bingöl C, Schuch B. Self-mutilation in adolescence as addictive behaviour. *Wien Klin Wochenschr* 1996;108(3):82–4.

138. Nixon MK, Cloutier PF, Aggarwal S. Affect regulation and addictive aspects of repetitive self-injury in hospitalized adolescents. *J Am Acad Child Adolesc Psychiatry* 2002;41(11):1333–41.

139. Slap G, Goodman E, Huang B. Adoption as a risk factor for attempted suicide during adolescence. *Pediatrics* 2001;108(2):E30.

140. Laukkanen E, Honkalampi K, Hintikka J, *et al.* Suicidal ideation among help-seeking adolescents: association with a negative self-image. *Arch Suicide Res* 2005;9(1):45–55.

141. Nock MK, Wedig MM, Holmberg EB, Hooley JM. The emotion reactivity scale: development, evaluation, and relation to self-injurious thoughts and behaviors. *Behav Ther* 2008;39(2):107–16.

142. Najmi S, Wegner DM, Nock MK. Thought suppression and self-injurious thoughts and behaviors. *Behav Res Ther* 2007;45(8):1957–65.

143. Brent DA. Risk factors for adolescent suicide and suicidal behavior: mental and substance abuse disorders, family environmental factors, and life stress. *Suicide Life Threat Behav* 1995;25(Suppl):52–63.

144. Brent DA, Bridge J, Johnson BA, Connolly J. Suicidal behavior runs in families. A controlled family study of adolescent suicide victims. *Arch Gen Psychiatry* 1996;53(12):1145–52.

145. Gould MS, Fisher P, Parides M, *et al.* Psychosocial risk factors of child and adolescent completed suicide. *Arch Gen Psychiatry* 1996;53(12):1155–62.

146. King RA, Schwab-Stone M, Flisher AJ, et al. Psychosocial and risk behavior correlates of youth suicide attempts and suicidal ideation. *J Am Acad Child Adolesc Psychiatry* 2001;40(7):837–46.

147. Brent DA, Melhem N. Familial transmission of suicidal behavior. *Psychiatr Clin North Am* 2008;31(2):157–77.

148. Brent DA, Mann JJ. Family genetic studies, suicide, and suicidal behavior. *Am J Med Genet C Semin Med Genet* 2005;133C(1):13–24.

149. Brent DA, Oquendo M, Birmaher B, et al. Familial pathways to early-onset suicide attempt: risk for suicidal behavior in offspring of mood-disordered suicide attempters. *Arch Gen Psychiatry* 2002;59(9):801–7.

150. Goodwin RD, Beautrais AL, Fergusson DM. Familial transmission of suicidal ideation and suicide attempts: evidence from a general population sample. *Psychiatry Res* 2004;126(2):159–65.

151. Agerbo E, Nordentoft M, Mortensen PB. Familial, psychiatric, and socioeconomic risk factors for suicide in young people: nested case-control study. *BMJ* 2002;325(7355):74.

152. Brent DA, Perper JA, Moritz G, et al. Familial risk factors for adolescent suicide: a case-control study. *Acta Psychiatr Scand* 1994;89(1):52–8.

153. Groholt B, Ekeberg Ø, Haldorsen T. Adolescent suicide attempters: what predicts future suicidal acts? *Suicide Life Threat Behav* 2006;36(6):638–50.

154. Wedig MM, Nock MK. Parental expressed emotion and adolescent self-injury. *J Am Acad Child Adolesc Psychiatry* 2007;46(9):1171–8.

155. Lewinsohn PM, Rohde P, Seeley JR. Adolescent suicidal ideation and attempts: Prevalence, risk factors, and clinical implications. *Clin Psychol Sci Prac* 1996:3(1):25–36.

156. Pfeffer CR, Karus D, Siegel K, Jiang H. Child survivors of parental death from cancer or suicide: depressive and behavioral outcomes. *Psychooncology* 2000;9(1):1–10.

157. Cerel J, Fristad MA, Weller EB, Weller RA. Suicide-bereaved children and adolescents: a controlled longitudinal examination. *J Am Acad Child Adolesc Psychiatry*. 1999;38(6): 672–9.

158. Cerel J, Fristad MA, Verducci J, et al. Childhood bereavement: psychopathology in the 2 years postparental death. *J Am Acad Child Adolesc Psychiatry* 2006;45(6):681–90.

159. Melhem NM, Walker M, Moritz G, Brent DA. Antecedents and sequelae of sudden parental death in offspring and surviving caregivers. *Arch Pediatr Adolesc Med* 2008;162(5):403–10.

160. Shaffer D, Fisher P, Hicks RH, et al. Sexual orientation in adolescents who commit suicide. *Suicide Life Threat Behav* 1995;25 (Suppl):64–71.

161. Eisenberg ME, Resnick MD. Suicidality among gay, lesbian and bisexual youth: the role of protective factors. *J Adolesc* Health 2006;39(5):662–8.

162. Fergusson DM, Horwood LJ, Beautrais AL. Is sexual orientation related to mental health problems and suicidality in young people? *Arch Gen Psychiatry* 1999;56(10):876–80.

163. Fleming TM, Merry SN, Robinson EM, et al. Self-reported suicide attempts and associated risk and protective factors among secondary school students in New Zealand. *Aust N Z J Psychiatry* 2007;41(3):213–21.

164. Garofalo R, Wolf C, Wissow LS, et al. Sexual orientation and risk of suicide attempts among a representative sample of youth. *Arch Pediatr Adolesc Med* 1999;153(5):487–493.

165. Remafedi G, French S, Story M, et al. The relationship between suicide risk and sexual orientation: results of a population-based study. *Am J Public Health* 1998;88(1):57–60.

166. Russell ST, Joyner K. Adolescent sexual orientation and suicide risk: evidence from a national study. *Am J Public Health* 2001;91(8):1276–81.

167. D'Augelli AR, Hershberger SL, Pilkington NW. Suicidality patterns and sexual orientation-related factors among lesbian, gay, and bisexual youths. *Suicide Life Threat Behav* 2001;31(3):250–64.

168. D'Augelli AR, Grossman AH, Salter NP, *et al.* Predicting the suicide attempts of lesbian, gay, and bisexual youth. *Suicide Life Threat Behav* 2005;35(6):646–60

169. Hershberger SL, Pilkington NW, D'Augelli AR. Predictors of suicide attempts among gay, lesbian, and bisexual youth. *J Adolesc Res* 1997;12(4):477–97.

170. Bergen HA, Martin G, Richardson AS, *et al.* Sexual abuse and suicidal behavior: a model constructed from a large community sample of adolescents. *J Am Acad Child Adolesc Psychiatry* 2003;42(11):1301–9.

171. Eisenberg ME, Ackard DM, Resnick MD. Protective factors and suicide risk in adolescents with a history of sexual abuse. *J Pediatr* 2007;151(5):482–7.

172. Fergusson DM, Boden JM, Horwood LJ. Exposure to childhood sexual and physical abuse and adjustment in early adulthood. *Child Abuse Negl* 2008;32(6):607–19.

173. Fergusson DM, Lynskey MT. Physical punishment/maltreatment during childhood and adjustment in young adulthood. *Child Abuse Negl* 1997;21(7):617–30.

174. Grilo CM, Sanislow C, Fehon DC, *et al.* Psychological and behavioral functioning in adolescent psychiatric inpatients who report histories of childhood abuse. *Am J Psychiatry* 1999;156(4):538–43.

175. Joiner TE, Jr, Sachs-Ericsson NJ, Wingate LR, *et al.* Childhood physical and sexual abuse and lifetime number of suicide attempts: a persistent and theoretically important relationship. *Behav Res Ther* 2007;45(3):539–47.

176. Lynskey MT, Fergusson DM. Factors protecting against the development of adjustment difficulties in young adults exposed to childhood sexual abuse. *Child Abuse Negl* 1997;21(12):1177–90.

177. Salzinger S, Rosario M, Feldman RS, Ng-Mak DS. Adolescent suicidal behavior: associations with preadolescent physical abuse and selected risk and protective factors. *J Am Acad Child Adolesc Psychiatry* 2007;46(7):859–66.

178. Brodsky BS, Mann JJ, Stanley B, *et al.* Familial transmission of suicidal behavior: factors mediating the relationship between childhood abuse and offspring suicide attempts. *J Clin Psychiatry* 2008;69(4):584–96.

179. Glassman LH, Weierich MR, Hooley JM, *et al.* Child maltreatment, non-suicidal self-injury, and the mediating role of self-criticism. *Behav Res Ther* 2007;45(10):2483–90.

180. Hacker KA, Suglia SF, Fried LE, *et al.* Developmental differences in risk factors for suicide attempts between ninth and eleventh graders. *Suicide Life Threat Behav* 2006;36(2):154–66.

181. Brunstein Klomek A, Marrocco F, Kleinman M, *et al.* Bullying, depression, and suicidality in adolescents. *J Am Acad Child Adolesc Psychiatry* 2007;46(1):40–9.

182. Lewinsohn PM, Rohde P, Seeley JR. Psychosocial characteristics of adolescents with a history of suicide attempt. *J Am Acad Child Adolesc Psychiatry* 1993;32(1):60–8.

183. Barker ED, Arseneault L, Brendgen M, *et al.* Joint development of bullying and victimization in adolescence: relations to delinquency and self-harm. *J Am Acad Child Adolesc Psychiatry* 2008;47(9):1030–8.

184. Klomek AB, Marrocco F, Kleinman M, *et al.* Peer victimization, depression, and suicidiality in adolescents. *Suicide Life Threat Behav* 2008;38(2):166–80

185. Resnick MD, Bearman PS, Blum RW, *et al.* Protecting adolescents from harm. Findings from the National Longitudinal Study on Adolescent Health. *JAMA* 1997;278(10):823–32.

186. Brent DA, Moritz G, Bridge J, *et al.* Long-term impact of exposure to suicide: a three-year controlled follow-up. *J Am Acad Child Adolesc Psychiatry* 1996;35(5):646–53.

187. Prinstein MJ, Boergers J, Spirito A. Adolescents' and their friends' health-risk behavior: factors that alter or add to peer influence. *J Pediatr Psychol* 2001;26(5):287–98.

188. Brent DA, Kerr MM, Goldstein C, *et al.* An outbreak of suicide and suicidal behavior in a high school. *J Am Acad Child Adolesc Psychiatry* 1989;28(6):918–24.

189. Gould MS, Wallenstein S, Kleinman M. Time-space clustering of teenage suicide. *Am J Epidemiol* 1990;131(1):71–8.

190. Gould MS, Wallenstein S, Kleinman MH, *et al.* Suicide clusters: an examination of age-specific effects. *Am J Public Health* 1990;80(2):211–2.

191. Gould MS, Petrie K, Kleinman MH, Wallenstein S. Clustering of attempted suicide: New Zealand national data. *Int J Epidemiol* 1994;23(6):1185–9.

192. Gould MS. Suicide and the media. *Ann N Y Acad Sci* 2001;932:200–21;

193. Hawton K, Townsend E, Deeks J, *et al.* Effects of legislation restricting pack sizes of paracetamol and salicylate on self poisoning in the United Kingdom: before and after study. *BMJ* 2001 May 19;322(7296):1203–7.

194. Hawton K, Simkin S, Deeks J, *et al.* UK legislation on analgesic packs: before and after study of long term effect on poisonings. *BMJ* 2004;329(7474):1076.

195. Brent DA, Perper JA, Moritz G, *et al.* Firearms and adolescent suicide. A community case-control study. *Am J Dis Child* 1993;147(10):1066–71.

196. Ajdacic-Gross V, Killias M, Hepp U, *et al.* Changing times: a longitudinal analysis of international firearm suicide data. *Am J Public Health* 2006;96(10):1752–5.

197. Beautrais AL, Fergusson DM, Horwood LJ. Firearms legislation and reductions in firearm-related suicide deaths in New Zealand. *Aust N Z J Psychiatry* 2006;40(3):253–9.

198. Goldston DB, Molock SD, Whitbeck LB, *et al.* Cultural considerations in adolescent suicide prevention and psychosocial treatment. *Am Psychol* 2008;63(1):14–31.

199. Hilton SC, Fellingham GW, Lyon JL. Suicide rates and religious commitment in young adult males in Utah. *Am J Epidemiol* 2002;155(5):413–9.

200. Siegrist M. Church attendance, denomination, and suicide ideology. *J Soc Psychol* 1996;136(5):559–66.

201. Zhang J, Jin S. Determinants of suicide ideation: a comparison of Chinese and American college students. *Adolescence* 1996;31(122):451–67.

CHAPTER 6

EFFECTIVE INTERVENTIONS

Dennis Ougrin

Introduction

The importance of treatment for adolescents presenting with self-harm has traditionally been underpinned by the link between self-harm and suicide: prior self-harm is estimated to have occurred in 25–33 per cent of all completed suicides, with the risk of completed suicide being higher for boys (30-fold) than for girls (threefold).[1] In recent years, however, the impact of self-harm on a range of psychosocial outcomes has been documented. Adolescents who self-harm are at a greater risk of substance misuse and a range of psychiatric disorders,[2] as well as psychosocial adversity in general.[3] Nonetheless the risk of suicide is one of the most important factors to bear in mind when treating this group and suicide prevention is among the main goals.

There are two main methods for suicide prevention: population-based strategies and intervention strategies in high-risk groups.

To date, the population-based strategies that have shown promise in reducing suicide can be summarised as follows:[4]

1. restriction of access to means to suicide. For example, alcohol,[5] firearms,[6] toxic over-the-counter medicines,[7-9] carbon monoxide[9-11] and access to suicide hot spots;[12-15]
2. issuing media guidelines on reporting suicides;[16]
3. psychoeducation;[17,18]
4. training primary care workers in the screening and detection of patients with a high risk of suicide.[19,20]

The rest of this chapter will discuss treatment strategies aimed towards adolescents who self-harm, one of the key target groups for the prevention of suicide.

It is especially important to clearly define self-harm when reviewing treatment studies. As previously indicated, in this text we will use the definition of self-harm as self-poisoning or self-injury, irrespective of the apparent purpose of the act,[21] thus capturing a wide range of self-harming behaviour. Even with this broad definition, there is an ongoing debate in terms of where to draw the line between self-harm and other potentially harmful behaviours like drug and alcohol misuse at one end of the spectrum and the self-harm seen in neurodevelopmental conditions at the other. Another important question is whether suicidal thinking is a legitimate target for intervention if one were to accept it as a point on the continuum of suicidality. For the purposes of this chapter we will not include studies that consider adolescents presenting with alcohol intoxication if self-harm/suicidality was an exclusion criterion[22] and the studies primarily concerned with self-harm in the population of those with severe to profound learning disability (mental retardation).[23,24]

It seems paradoxical that despite self-harm clearly being much more prevalent in adolescence, and reducing considerably by early adulthood,[25] there are many more controlled intervention studies aimed at self-harm reduction in adults[26–38] or mixed populations with adolescents comprising only a minority of the participants.[36,39]

This chapter mainly focuses on the published randomised controlled trials (RCTs) of therapeutic interventions specifically targeting adolescents with self-harm behaviours. At present there are eight randomised studies published meeting these criteria. They will be examined one by one, starting with those showing statistically significant improvements with respect to self-harm.[40]

Developmental group psychotherapy

In a study by Wood et al.[40] 63 participants (mean age 14 years, range 12–16 years, 78 per cent female) were allocated to either developmental group therapy or standard care. Group therapy involved a minimum of six sessions, after which participants were free to choose how much longer they remained in a long-term support group. Apart from group treatment there was an option of individual top-up sessions, broadly along cognitive–behavioural therapy (CBT) lines. At 29 weeks follow-up there was a significant difference favouring group therapy over standard aftercare with respect to reducing the likelihood of engaging in two or more episodes of self-harm (relative risk = 0.19; 95% CI 0.05–0.81). There was also a positive effect on a range of behavioural problems.

The authors included a broad range of self-harm behaviours in line with Hawton's definition of self-harm,[21] as adopted by the National Institute for Clinical Excellence (NICE), but excluded accidental ingestion of substances, the use of substances to obtain a 'high' or pure alcohol intoxication.

The intervention was manualised and included elements of a broad range of therapies including problem-solving, cognitive–behavioural interventions, dialectical behaviour therapy and psychodynamic group psychotherapy. There were two groups running in parallel continuously, one acute and one long-term support, and the adolescents did not have to wait to join either. In addition some of the adolescents attended individual sessions with the group therapists.

This study has many strong points. First, relatively good engagement with treatment was achieved in this study: only 16 of the 80 eligible adolescents refused to participate and 64 were randomised into two groups with 32 subjects in each. Most patients completed four or more sessions of either the intervention or the routine care, 23/32 and 19/32 respectively. Second, the treatment allocation was random and concealed, there was a true intention to treat analysis (i.e. in that all adolescents were analysed in the groups they had been randomised to, not just those that completed the treatment) and the outcome data were available for 98 per cent of the adolescents. Third, the study reported a range of outcomes relevant to patients' wellbeing. Fourth, the study was pragmatic in that broad inclusion criteria were used and the participants were roughly representative of routine clinical care, making results more generalisable. Finally, this manualised intervention was administered by only two professionals, making it potentially attractive from a service planning point of view.

Perhaps the most important disadvantage of this study is its poor applicability in other settings. Although the intervention was manualised, both therapists had extensive previous training and presumably were familiar with the principles of a broad range of therapies. This cannot be expected from clinicians delivering care in other services. In addition, no information was provided about the length and the nature of training required to provide this intervention. The authors did not specify the rationale for choosing the main outcome measure (i.e. engaging in two or more episodes of self-harm during follow-up) – from the introduction to the article it appears that repetition of self-harm and depressive symptoms were the original primary outcome measures. The authors reported that there were no differences between the groups in terms of depressive symptoms or suicidal thinking. The reported reduction in self-harm does not appear to hold if the absolute number of self-harm episodes is taken into account (intervention mean = 0.6, 95% CI 0.3–0.9 vs routine care mean = 1.8, 95% CI 0.6–3.0). It would appear from the overlapping confidence intervals that the difference was not statistically significant (although this difference may well be clinically significant).

Nonetheless, this study reported the most encouraging results in the treatment of adolescents with self-harm to date. Developmental group therapy is tentatively recommended by NICE.[21] The study also challenged a widely held assumption that treating adolescents in groups may cause more harm than benefit.

A larger study from the same research group is under way and replication of the findings from independent researchers would be much welcomed, coupled with a coherent system for training and dissemination of the treatment, should the results of the definitive study prove similarly positive.

Multisystemic therapy

Multisystemic therapy (MST) is a modification of family therapy that takes into account multiple systems that the family and the adolescents interact with. The main aim of the therapy is effective parenting skills, primarily targeted at engaging young people with pro-social activities and disengaging from antisocial ones, removing potential methods of suicide and monitoring and support of the young people by responsible adults. Apart from the family, community, school and peer systems are targeted. The therapy is intensive (contact could be daily) and time limited (3–6 months). Contacts are made in adolescents' homes and the average caseload of the therapists is low (four to six families).

In a random allocation trial, MST was studied in a sample of adolescents referred to an emergency department and authorised for psychiatric admission ($n = 156$, age 10–17 years, average age 12.9 years, 65 per cent male, 65 per cent African American), 51 per cent of these young people were classified as suicidal (suicidal ideation or attempt) and the rest had a variety of severe psychiatric problems. These young people were randomised to either MST or hospitalisation. Based on youth reports, MST was significantly more effective than emergency hospitalisation at decreasing rates of attempted suicide at 1-year follow-up. Multisystemic therapy did not have any differential effect on depression, hopelessness or suicidal ideation.

This study is important in several ways. First, it studies a sample of economically disadvantaged adolescents from a predominantly ethnic minority background. This is a significantly under-researched group, possibly having important differential responses to psychotherapy. Second, the study uses sound methodology with concealed allocation to treatment conditions and high retention rates (97.5 per cent). Only 17 families refused to participate in the study and 160 consented, 74 of the 79 families randomised to the MST condition completed a full course of treatment, with an average duration of 127 days (SD = 32 days).

Finally the study used well-validated measures of both suicidal behaviour and ideation as well as both youth and parent reports. As in the Wood et al.[40] study, the biggest problem with this study is applicability, but generalisability is also an important issue. On one hand MST requires extensive training and resources, rarely available in community child psychiatry services. On the other hand, the young people studied presented with a mixture of psychiatric problems and only a minority had self-harm as a presenting problem. In addition, the average age of the participants (12.9 years) was unusually young for studies of adolescents with self-harm. It was unfortunate that the proportion of the young people with both suicidal ideation and a history of self-harm was greater in the MST group than in the hospitalisation (control) group. As the proportion of the young people reporting self-harm at 1-year follow-up did not differ between the arms of the study – 4 per cent each on the Youth Risk Behavior Survey (YRBS) attempted suicide measure – this does not allow for exclusion of a regression to the mean as a possible explanation for the reduction of self-harm in the MST arm from baseline. The interpretation of the findings is further confounded by the fact that 44 per cent of the youth in the MST arm were hospitalised in the course of the trial. The authors did not explicitly state which outcome measures they considered to be primary and they also created dichotomised outcome measures (i.e. suicidal or not, having attempted self-harm or not) not pre-specified a priori. Finally, comparing MST with hospitalisation may give an important insight into the choice of management strategy for acutely distressed adolescents. It does not necessarily help in deciding on the best strategy for the outpatient management of these young people.

The rest of the RCTs in this patient group have not shown positive results on primary outcome measures. They are reviewed below.

Family therapy[41,42] was delivered by therapeutic social workers to adolescents who poisoned themselves ($n = 162$, age <16 years). The therapy was carried out at home and consisted of a single assessment session and four treatment sessions. The main focus of the treatment was on problem solving. There were no differences between the groups with respect to the main outcome measures which included suicidal ideation. The treatment resulted in decreased suicidal ideation only in a subgroup of adolescents without depression. The study also found improved parent-rated satisfaction and better engagement with family therapy than with treatment as usual.

In a study of a Youth-Nominated Support Team for Suicidal Adolescents,[43] a social intervention was compared with treatment as usual in a sample of suicidal adolescents ($n = 289$, age 12–17 years). The intervention involved youths nominating up to four important people from their family, school, community or peer group. These individuals were then trained in understanding and supporting the young people and were encouraged to establish weekly contact with the adolescent. There were no differences between the groups on any of the main outcome measures including suicidal ideation and attempts. Some positive impact was shown on suicidal ideation and depression-related functioning in a subgroup consisting of girls alone.

Spirito et al.[44] tested standard disposition planning (routine discharge) versus a 1-hour compliance enhancement intervention using a problem-solving format in a sample of adolescents ($n = 63$, age 12–18 years) who presented to hospital following a suicide attempt. Adolescents in the compliance enhancement group were then regularly contacted by phone to encourage attendance. There was no significant improvement in the number of sessions attended (7.7 sessions compared with 6.4 sessions) in the main analysis. A statistically significant improvement in the number of sessions attended was reported after adjusting for barriers to services (mean = 8.4 vs 5.8 sessions). No suicide-related outcomes at follow-up were reported in this study.

Skills-based treatment versus supportive relationship treatment was compared in a study of 39 adolescents (age 12–17 years) and their parents who presented to a hospital after a suicide attempt. Skills-based treatment focused on teaching skills in problem solving and affect regulation based on cognitive–behavioural ideas. Supportive relationship treatment comprised unstructured supportive sessions without specific skills training. Both treatments were delivered in a combination of up to 14 individual and family sessions. There were no differences found between the treatment conditions on any of the main outcome measures, including suicidal thinking and behaviour. The authors reported good adherence to treatment and improvements in suicidal ideation and depressive mood in both arms of the study.

Another trial compared up to 24 sessions of cognitive analytic therapy (CAT) versus manualised good clinical care in a referred outpatient sample of 86 adolescents (age 15–18 years) meeting between two and nine diagnostic criteria for borderline personality disorder. Over 70 per cent of the adolescents engaged in self-harm regularly at baseline. There were no differences between the groups in the main outcome measures that included self-harm behaviours: both groups improved significantly. Adolescents in the CAT arm showed a more rapid improvement.

The issue of tokens allowing young people hospital readmission plus usual management was compared with usual management alone in a sample of 105 adolescents (age 12–16 years) who presented to the emergency department following a suicide attempt.[45] No statistically significant differences were found between the two arms in the rates of further suicide attempts. In the experimental group only three adolescents made further suicide attempts in the following year and five made use of their tokens to gain hospital admission, while in the control group seven made further suicide attempts.

Dialectical behaviour therapy

There are a number of other therapeutic modalities that have recently been evaluated and show promise in the treatment of adolescent self-harm. However, they have not been subject to rigorous testing in random allocation trials. Dialectical behaviour therapy (DBT) has been tested in several RCTs in adult populations.[26,27,46] primarily involving female patients with borderline personality disorder. Dialectical behaviour therapy was also piloted in adolescents in uncontrolled studies with positive results on measures of depression, hopelessness, episodes of self-harm and an improvement in general functioning.[47–49] In controlled studies the results were somewhat more mixed. No significant differences were noted on measures of parasuicidal behaviour, depressive symptoms and suicidal ideation[50] or suicidal attempts.[47] However, DBT has been shown to significantly reduce behavioural incidents during inpatient admissions.[50] When compared with individual supportive-psychodynamic therapy plus weekly family therapy (designated as treatment as usual) the DBT group had significantly fewer psychiatric hospitalisations and a significantly higher rate of treatment completion.[47]

Interpersonal psychotherapy

Interpersonal psychotherapy (IPT) is a well recognised treatment for adolescent depression[51-53] as well as being a possible preventative strategy.[54] Interpersonal psychotherapy has been tried in an open trial in adolescents ($n = 10$, age 14–18 years) with a history of self-harm and a diagnosis of bipolar disorder, leading to a reduction of suicidality, non-suicidal self-injurious behaviour, emotional dysregulation and depressive symptoms.[55]

Cognitive–behaviour therapy

Cognitive–behaviour therapy is also a well recognised treatment for adolescent depression,[56] although the early large effect sizes have not been sustained in recent trials.[57-59] It may also be a possible preventative strategy against depression.[53] In multicentre trials the effect of CBT on suicidality in depressed adolescents has been controversial. In the Treatment for Adolescents with Depression Study (TADS), 439 patients aged 12–17 years with major depressive disorder were randomly allocated to one of four treatment arms, each lasting 12 weeks: fluoxetine alone (10–40 mg per day); CBT alone; CBT with fluoxetine; or placebo.[58,59] The CBT arm was associated with a greater reduction in suicidal thinking than either fluoxetine alone or a combination of fluoxetine and CBT. Patients treated in all arms showed a reduction in suicidal ideation across the trial. Cognitive–behavioural therapy has also been tried in adolescents with both suicidal thoughts and substance misuse problems, leading to an improvement in both at follow-up with individual face-to-face aftercare.[60-62]

In the Treatment of SSRI-Resistant Depression in Adolescents (TORDIA) trial[63] and in the Adolescent Depression Antidepressant and Psychotherapy Trial (ADAPT),[57] CBT did not have a protective effect on suicidal ideation or self-harm. These results are reflected in a meta-analysis of adolescent studies that does not support the efficacy of CBT to reduce suicidal behaviour in adolescents,[64] despite the meta-analysis including DBT and non-randomised studies.

Finally, a definitive study on the treatment of adolescents with suicide attempts that compares a number of psychopharmacological agents with and without CBT, Treatment of Adolescent Suicide Attempters (TASA), has been plagued with difficulties,[65] leading some researchers to question if randomised designs are a feasible format for studying interventions in this patient group.[66]

Emergency department interventions

A specialised emergency room programme for adolescent attempters has demonstrated increased adherence to treatment aftercare,[67-70] although the numbers of sessions attended increased only marginally (5.4 vs 4.7). The programme included an intervention from an on-call family therapist, a soap opera video regarding suicidality and additional staff training. The participants were 140 females (age 12–18 years) of Hispanic origin. Other authors did not find brief psychotherapeutic compliance-enhancement intervention effective at increasing engagement with follow-up.[71] The studies designed to evaluate the effectiveness of emergency department-based interventions aimed at reducing adolescents' access to means of self-harm reported both positive[72] and discouraging[73] results. An intervention designed to avert inpatient hospitalisation, the Systemic Crisis Intervention Programme, was tested in a sample of 47 adolescents (age 7–19 years) and showed favourable results in terms of self-harm behaviour and hospitalisation, as well as improvement in family functioning and the subjects' behavioural disturbance.

How do clinical guidelines interpret this evidence? British and American guidelines take diametrically opposite views. The American Academy of Child and Adolescent Psychiatry's Practice Parameters recommend considering all of these therapies: CBT, IPT, DBT, psychodynamic therapy and family therapy; however, British guidelines take a conservative stance with only developmental group psychotherapy for repeat self-harmers being recommended for consideration.

At present, studies of pharmacological interventions are lagging behind studies of psychotherapeutic interventions. There are no current RCTs examining the impact of psychopharmacological agents on self-harm in adolescents, although in adults a range of agents have been evaluated.[27,74–82] There has been a recent shift from the traditional focus on selective serotonin reuptake inhibitors (SSRIs) towards mood stabilising and antipsychotic agents in the adult literature.[77]

One area of particular controversy in child and adolescent psychiatry is the association between suicidality and the use of SSRIs. In October 2004 the American regulatory agency for medicines, the Food and Drug Administration (FDA), mandated manufacturers to use black boxes on SSRI packets warning of an increased risk of suicidality in paediatric patients. The warnings about a possible association were first issued in October 2003. By February 2005 the FDA had provided specific language for the warning and required a patient medication guide. This led to a decrease in the prescription rates in this age group.[83] However, contrary to predictions, the suicide rate among adolescents in the USA increased in both 2004 and 2005.[84] Although no causality can be assumed, many researchers propose that adequate treatment of paediatric depression may have been compromised by the FDA action.

Was the FDA right in raising this concern? The FDA commissioned a meta-analysis that pooled data from RCTs comparing SSRIs and Venlafaxine with placebo for the following indications: major depressive disorder (MDD, 16 trials), obsessive–compulsive disorder (OCD, four trials), generalised anxiety disorder (two trials), social anxiety disorder (one trial), and attention-deficit/hyperactivity disorder (one trial). The primary model of meta-analysis reported was the fixed-effects model. The overall suicidality risk ratio for SSRIs versus placebo in depression trials was 1.66 (95 per cent, CI 1.02–2.68) and for all drugs across all indications was 1.95 (95 per cent, CI 1.28–2.98). In other words, the use of antidepressants was associated with a twofold (4 per cent vs 2 per cent) increase in the risk of suicidal thoughts and suicidal behaviour. The authors concluded that the use of antidepressant drugs in paediatric patients is associated with a modestly increased risk of suicidality.

However, a different meta-analysis using the random-effects model showed a smaller although still statistically significant overall risk ratio for suicidality 1.7 (CI 1.1–2.7)[85]. Breaking the data down according to the three main indications examined (MDD, OCD and non-OCD anxiety disorders) the authors showed a more favourable risk–benefit ratio with the use of SSRIs (and Venlafaxine) for each indication, with caveats that this ratio is inversely proportional to the age of subjects and is most favourable in non-OCD anxiety disorders.

Since the publication of both meta-analyses two multicentre studies have failed to show a statistically significant increase in the incidence of suicidality with SSRIs (and Venlafaxine) versus placebo-treated adolescents.[57,63]

Despite this, following the advice of the Committee on Safety of Medicines (CSM), the British equivalent of the FDA, the Medicines and Healthcare Products Regulatory Agency (MHRA) presently considers that only Fluoxetine has a favourable balance of risks and benefits in the treatment of child and adolescent depression. The European Medicines Evaluation Agency (EMEA) took a similar line suggesting SSRIs and SNRIs should generally not be used for treating depression in children. If they are used, patients should be carefully monitored for the appearance of any suicidality or violence.

These developments were reflected in the NICE guidelines on the management of depression[86] and self-harm.[21]

Summary

So what are clinicians to make of this? First, self-harm as a behaviour probably requires treatment in its own right, as addressing supposedly underlying psychiatric conditions does not seem to improve self-harm. Second, at present psychological treatments have more, albeit limited, evidence supporting their use than pharmacological agents. Third, there is no good reason to believe that a single intervention would be beneficial for all adolescents and it may be that different adolescents may respond to different interventions.

On the basis of the available evidence one might conclude that the optimal treatment for adolescents who self-harm should be conducted on an outpatient basis, have a group component and be done by a dedicated team that consists of therapists with low caseloads who have a mutual support structure.

As far as the possible targets for an intervention are concerned, these are likely to be specific to each individual and perhaps hierarchical. That is to say that many young people who self-harm recover with minimal or no support and many may benefit from simple behavioural or cognitive interventions. However, there is a group of young people who self-harm who undoubtedly have much greater needs and who require a form of highly specialised support. The targets for this group may include changes within multiple social systems that perpetuate self-harm, developing emotional regulation skills and improving interpersonal functioning. Dialectical behaviour therapy, IPT, MST or perhaps mentalisation-based therapy (MBT) may be options for these young people.

Finally it is worth noting that psychotherapy is a skill-based intervention, perhaps more akin to surgery than medication treatment. Adequate training and supervision of therapists is therefore the key to the successful delivery of treatment for self-harm.

References

1. Shaffer D, Gould MS, Fisher P, *et al*. Psychiatric diagnosis in child and adolescent suicide. *Arch Gen Psychiatry* 1996;53(4):339–48.
2. Steinhausen H-C, Bosiger R, Metzke CW. Stability, correlates, and outcome of adolescent suicidal risk. *J Child Psychol Psychiatry* 2006;47(7):713–22.
3. Harrington R, Pickles A, Aglan A, *et al*. Early adult outcomes of adolescents who deliberately poisoned themselves. *J Am Acad Child Adolesc Psychiatry* 2006;45(3):337–45.
4. Mann JJ, Apter A, Bertolote J, *et al*. Suicide prevention strategies: a systematic review. *JAMA* 2005;294(16):2064–74.
5. Varnik A, Kolves K, Vali M, *et al*. Do alcohol restrictions reduce suicide mortality? *Addiction* 2007;102(2):251–6.
6. Kapusta ND, Etzersdorfer E, Krall C, Sonneck G. Firearm legislation reform in the European Union: Impact on firearm availability, firearm suicide and homicide rates in Austria. *Br J Psychiatry* 2007;191(3):253–7.
7. Hawkins LC, Edwards JN, Dargan PI. Impact of restricting paracetamol pack sizes on paracetamol poisoning in the United Kingdom: a review of the literature. *Drug Saf* 2007;30(6):465–79.
8. Hughes B, Durran A, Langford NJ, Mutimer D. Paracetamol poisoning – impact of pack size restrictions. *J Clin Pharm Ther* 2003;28(4):307–10.
9. Nordentoft M, Qin P, Helweg-Larsen K, Juel K. Restrictions in means for suicide: an effective tool in preventing suicide: the Danish experience. *Suicide Life Threat Behav* 2007;37(6):688–97.
10. Clarke RV, Lester D. Detoxification of motor vehicle exhaust and suicide. *Psychol Rep* 1986 Dec;59(3):1034.
11. Nordentoft M. Prevention of suicide and attempted suicide in Denmark. Epidemiological studies of suicide and intervention studies in selected risk groups. Dan Med Bull 2007;54(4):306–69.
12. Beautrais A. Suicide by jumping: A review of research and prevention strategies. *Crisis* 2007;28(Suppl 1):58–63.
13. Gunnell D, Nowers M. Suicide by jumping. *Acta Psychiatr Scand* 1997;96(1):1–6.
14. Pelletier AR. Preventing suicide by jumping: The effect of a bridge safety fence. *Inj Prev* 2007;13(1):57–9.
15. Reisch T, Schuster U, Michel K. Suicide by jumping and accessibility of bridges: results from a national survey in Switzerland. *Suicide Life Threat Behav* 2007;37(6):681–7.

16. Sonneck G, Etzersdorfer E, Nagel-Kuess S. Imitative suicide on the Viennese subway. *Soc Sci Med* 1994;38(3):453–7.

17. Aseltine RH, Jr, DeMartino R. An outcome evaluation of the SOS Suicide Prevention Program. *Am J Public Health* 2004;94(3):446–51.

18. Aseltine RH, Jr, James A, Schilling EA, *et al.* Evaluating the SOS suicide prevention program: a replication and extension. *BMC Public Health* 2007;7:161.

19. Rutz W, von Knorring L, Walinder J. Frequency of suicide on Gotland after systematic postgraduate education of general practitioners. *Acta Psychiatr Scand* 1989;80(2):151–4.

20. Beautrais A, Fergusson D, Coggan C, *et al.* Effective strategies for suicide prevention in New Zealand: a review of the evidence. *N Z Med J* 2007;120(1251):U2459.

21. National Collaborating Centre for Mental Health. Self-*harm: the short-term physical and psychological management and secondary prevention of self-harm in primary and secondary care.* Clinical Guideline 16. London: Gaskell & British Psychological Society; 2004.

22. Spirito A, Monti PM, Barnett NP, *et al.* A randomized clinical trial of a brief motivational intervention for alcohol-positive adolescents treated in an emergency department. *J Pediatr* 2004;145(3):396–402.

23. Petty J, Oliver C. Self-injurious behaviour in individuals with intellectual disabilities. *Curr Opin Psychiatry* 2005;18(5):484–9.

24. Symons FJ, Thompson A, Rodriguez MC. Self-injurious behavior and the efficacy of naltrexone treatment: a quantitative synthesis. *Ment Retard Dev Disabil Res Rev* 2004;10(3):193–200.

25. Favazza AR. The coming of age of self-mutilation. *J Nerv Ment Dis* 1998;186(5):259–68.

26. Linehan MM, Comtois KA, Murray AM, *et al.* Two-year randomized controlled trial and follow-up of dialectical behavior therapy vs therapy by experts for suicidal behaviors and borderline personality disorder. [Erratum appears in *Arch Gen Psychiatry* 2007;64(12): 1401]. *Arch Gen Psychiatry* 2006;63(7):757–66.

27. Linehan MM, McDavid JD, Brown MZ, *et al.* Olanzapine plus dialectical behavior therapy for women with high irritability who meet criteria for borderline personality disorder: a double-blind, placebo-controlled pilot study. *J Clin Psychiatry* 2008;69(6):999–1005.

28. Linehan MM, Schmidt H, 3rd, Dimeff LA, *et al.* Dialectical behavior therapy for patients with borderline personality disorder and drug-dependence. *Am J Addict* 1999;8(4):279–92.

29. Bateman A, Fonagy P. Effectiveness of partial hospitalization in the treatment of borderline personality disorder: a randomized controlled trial. *Am J Psychiatry* 1999 Oct;156(10): 1563–9.

30. Bateman A, Fonagy P. Treatment of borderline personality disorder with psychoanalytically oriented partial hospitalization: an 18-month follow-up. *Am J Psychiatry* 2001;158(1): 36–42.

31. Bateman A, Fonagy P. 8-year follow-up of patients treated for borderline personality disorder: mentalization-based treatment versus treatment as usual. *Am J Psychiatry* 2008;165(5):631–8.

32. Bennewith O, Stocks N, Gunnell D, *et al.* General practice based intervention to prevent repeat episodes of deliberate self-harm: cluster randomised controlled trial. *BMJ* 2002;324(7348):1254–7.

33. Tyrer P, Thompson S, Schmidt U, *et al.* Randomized controlled trial of brief cognitive behaviour therapy versus treatment as usual in recurrent deliberate self-harm: the POPMACT study [See comment.] *Psychol Med* 2003;33(6):969–76.

34. Vaiva G, Ducrocq F, Meyer P, *et al.* Effect of telephone contact on further suicide attempts in patients discharged from an emergency department: randomised controlled study. *BMJ* 2006;**332**(7552):1241–5.

35. Brown GK, Ten Have T, Henriques GR, *et al.* Cognitive therapy for the prevention of suicide attempts: a randomized controlled trial. *JAMA* 2005;**294**(5):563–70.

36. Carter GL, Clover K, Whyte IM, *et al.* Postcards from the EDge project: randomised controlled trial of an intervention using postcards to reduce repetition of hospital treated deliberate self poisoning. *BMJ* 2005;**331**(7520):805.

37. Evans J, Evans M, Morgan HG, *et al.* Crisis card following self-harm: 12-month follow-up of a randomised controlled trial. *Br J Psychiatry* 2005;**187**:186–7.

38. Guthrie E, Kapur N, Mackway-Jones K, *et al.* Randomised controlled trial of brief psychological intervention after deliberate self poisoning *BMJ* 2001;**323**(7305):135–8.

39. Slee N, Garnefski N, van der Leeden R, *et al.* Cognitive-behavioural intervention for self-harm: randomised controlled trial. *Br J Psychiatry* 2008;**192**(3):202–11.

40. Wood A, Trainor G, Rothwell J, Moore A, Harrington R. Randomized trial of group therapy for repeated deliberate self-harm in adolescents. *J Am Acad Child Adolesc Psychiatry* 2001;**40**(11):1246–53.

41. Byford S, Harrington R, Torgerson D, *et al.* Cost-effectiveness analysis of a home-based social work intervention for children and adolescents who have deliberately poisoned themselves. Results of a randomised controlled trial. *Br J Psychiatry* 1999;**174**:56–62.

42. Harrington R, Kerfoot M, Dyer E, *et al.* Randomized trial of a home-based family intervention for children who have deliberately poisoned themselves. *J Am Acad Child Adolesc Psychiatry* 1998;**37**(5):512–8.

43. King CA, Kramer A, Preuss L, *et al.* Youth-nominated support team for suicidal adolescents (Version 1): a randomized controlled trial. *J Consult Clin Psychol* 2006;**74**(1):199–206.

44. Spirito A, Boergers J, Donaldson D, *et al.* An intervention trial to improve adherence to community treatment by adolescents after a suicide attempt. *J Am Acad Child Adolesc Psychiatry* 2002;**41**(4):435–42.

45. Cotgrove AJ, Zirinsky L, Black D, Weston D. Secondary prevention of attempted suicide in adolescence. *J Adolesc* 1995;**18**(5):569–77.

46. Verheul R, Van Den Bosch LM, Koeter MW, *et al.* Dialectical behaviour therapy for women with borderline personality disorder: 12-month, randomised clinical trial in the Netherlands [See comment.] *Br J Psychiatry* 2003;**182**:135–40.

47. Rathus JH, Miller AL. Dialectical behavior therapy adapted for suicidal adolescents. *Suicide Life Threat Behav* 2002;**32**(2):146–57.

48. Fleischhaker C, Munz M, Bohme R, *et al.* Dialectical behaviour therapy for adolescents (DBT-A) – a pilot study on the therapy of suicidal, parasuicidal, and self-injurious behaviour in female patients with a borderline disorder. *Z Kinder Jugendpsychiatr Psychother* 2006;**34**(1):15–27.

49. James AC, Taylor A, Winmill L, Alfoadari K. A preliminary community study of dialectical behaviour therapy (DBT) with adolescent females demonstrating persistent, deliberate self-harm (DSH). *Child and Adolescent Mental Health* 2008;**13**(3):148–52.

50. Katz LY, Cox BJ, Gunasekara S, Miller AL. Feasibility of dialectical behavior therapy for suicidal adolescent inpatients. *J Am Acad Child Adolesc Psychiatry* 2004;**43**(3):276–82.

51. Klomek AB, Mufson L. Interpersonal psychotherapy for depressed adolescents. *Child Adolesc Psychiatr Clin N Am* 2006;**15**(4):959–75, ix.

52. Mufson L, Dorta KP, Wickramaratne P, *et al.* A randomized effectiveness trial of

interpersonal psychotherapy for depressed adolescents. *Arch Gen Psychiatry* 2004;**61**(6):577–84.

53. Rossello J, Bernal G, Rivera-Medina C. Individual and group CBT and IPT for Puerto Rican adolescents with depressive symptoms. *Cultur Divers Ethnic Minor Psychol* 2008;**14**(3):234–45.

54. Horowitz JL, Garber J, Ciesla JA, *et al.* Prevention of depressive symptoms in adolescents: a randomized trial of cognitive-behavioral and interpersonal prevention programs. *J Consult Clin Psychol* 2007;**75**(5):693–706.

55. Goldstein TR, Axelson DA, Birmaher B, Brent DA. Dialectical behavior therapy for adolescents with bipolar disorder: a 1-year open trial. *J Am Acad Child Adolesc Psychiatry* 2007 Jul;**46**(7):820–30.

56. Klein JB, Jacobs RH, Reinecke MA. Cognitive-behavioral therapy for adolescent depression: a meta-analytic investigation of changes in effect-size estimates. *J Am Acad Child Adolesc Psychiatry* 2007;**46**(11):1403–13.

57. Goodyer I, Dubicka B, Wilkinson P, *et al.* Selective serotonin reuptake inhibitors (SSRIs) and routine specialist care with and without cognitive behaviour therapy in adolescents with major depression: randomised controlled trial. *BMJ* 2007;**335**(7611):142.

58. March J, Silva S, Petrycki S, Curry J, *et al.* Fluoxetine, cognitive-behavioral therapy, and their combination for adolescents with depression: Treatment for Adolescents With Depression Study (TADS) randomized controlled trial *JAMA* 2004;**292**(7):807–20.

59. March JS, Silva S, Petrycki S, *et al.* The Treatment for Adolescents With Depression Study (TADS): long-term effectiveness and safety outcomes. *Arch Gen Psychiatry* 2007;**64**(10):1132–43.

60. Kaminer Y, Burleson JA, Goldberger R, *et al.* Cognitive-behavioral coping skills and psychoeducation therapies for adolescent substance abuse. *J Nerv Ment Dis* 2002;**190**(11): 737–45.

61. Kaminer Y, Burleson JA, Goldston DB, *et al.* Suicidal ideation among adolescents with alcohol use disorders during treatment and aftercare. *Am J Addict* 2006;**15**(Suppl 1):43–9.

62. Kaminer Y, Napolitano C. Dial for therapy: aftercare for adolescent substance use disorders. *J Am Acad Child Adolesc Psychiatry* 2004;**43**(9):1171–4.

63. Brent D, Emslie G, Clarke G, *et al.* Switching to another SSRI or to venlafaxine with or without cognitive behavioral therapy for adolescents with SSRI-resistant depression: The TORDIA randomized controlled trial. *JAMA* 2008;**299**(8):901–13.

64. Tarrier N, Taylor K, Gooding P. Cognitive-behavioral interventions to reduce suicide behavior: a systematic review and meta-analysis. *Behav Modif* 2008;**32**(1):77–108.

65. NIH. *Treatment of adolescent suicide attempters* (TASA), 2008 [accessed 24 December 2008] Available from: http://www.clinicaltrials.gov/ct2/show/NCT00080158?term=tasa&rank=1.

66. Cwik MF, Walkup JT. Can randomized controlled trials be done with suicidal youths? *Int Rev Psychiatry* 2008;**20**(2):177–82.

67. Rotheram-Borus MJ, Piacentini J, Cantwell C, *et al.* The 18-month impact of an emergency room intervention for adolescent female suicide attempters. *J Consult Clin Psychol* 2000;**68**(6):1081–93.

68. Rotheram-Borus MJ, Piacentini J, Miller S, *et al.* Toward improving treatment adherence among adolescent suicide attempters. *Clin Child Psychol Psychiatry* 1996;**1**(1):99–108.

69. Rotheram-Borus MJ, Piacentini J, Van Rossem R, *et al.* Treatment adherence among Latina female adolescent suicide attempters. *Suicide Life Threat Behav* 1999;**29**(4):319–31.

70. Rotherham-Borus MJ, Piacentini J, Van Rossem R, *et al.* Enhancing treatment adherence

with a specialized emergency room program for adolescent suicide attempters. *J Am Acad Child Adolesc Psychiatry* 1996;35(5):654–63.

71. Zimmerman JK, Asnis GM, Schwartz BJ. Enhancing outpatient treatment compliance: a multifamily psychoeducational intake group. In: Zimmerman JK, Asnis GM, editors. *Treatment approaches with suicidal adolescents*. Oxford, UK: John Wiley & Sons; 1995: pp. 106–34.

72. Lerner MS, Clum GA. Treatment of suicide ideators: a problem-solving approach. *Beh Ther* 1990;21(4):403–11.

73. Brent DA, Baugher M, Birmaher B, *et al*. Compliance with recommendations to remove firearms in families participating in a clinical trial for adolescent depression. *J Am Acad Child Adolesc Psychiatry* 2000;39(10):1220–6.

74. Hallahan B, Hibbeln JR, Davis JM, *et al*. Omega-3 fatty acid supplementation in patients with recurrent self-harm. Single-centre double-blind randomised controlled trial. *Br J Psychiatry* 2007;190:118–22.

75. Meltzer HY, Alphs L, Green AI, *et al*. Clozapine treatment for suicidality in schizophrenia: International Suicide Prevention Trial (InterSePT). [Erratum appears in *Arch Gen Psychiatry* 2003;60(7):735.] *Arch Gen Psychiatry* 2003;60(1):82–91.

76. Nickel MK, Muehlbacher M, Nickel C, *et al*. Aripiprazole in the treatment of patients with borderline personality disorder: a double-blind, placebo-controlled study. *Am J Psychiatry* 2006;163(5):833–8.

77. Abraham PF, Calabrese JR. Evidenced-based pharmacologic treatment of borderline personality disorder: a shift from SSRIs to anticonvulsants and atypical antipsychotics? *J Affect Disord* 2008;111(1):21–30.

78. Bellino S, Paradiso E, Bogetto F. Efficacy and tolerability of pharmacotherapies for borderline personality disorder. *CNS Drugs* 2008;22(8):671–92.

79. Bogenschutz MP, George Nurnberg H. Olanzapine versus placebo in the treatment of borderline personality disorder. *J Clin Psychiatry* 2004;65(1):104–9.

80. Grootens KP, Verkes RJ. Emerging evidence for the use of atypical antipsychotics in borderline personality disorder. *Pharmacopsychiatry* 2005;38(1):20–3.

81. Simpson EB, Yen S, Costello E, *et al*. Combined dialectical behavior therapy and fluoxetine in the treatment of borderline personality disorder. *J Clin Psychiatry* 2004;65(3):379–85.

82. Zanarini MC, Frankenburg FR, Parachini EA. A preliminary, randomized trial of fluoxetine, olanzapine, and the olanzapine-fluoxetine combination in women with borderline personality disorder. *J Clin Psychiatry* 2004;65(7):903–7.

83. Libby AM, Brent DA, Morrato EH, *et al*. Decline in treatment of pediatric depression after FDA advisory on risk of suicidality with SSRIs. *Am J Psychiatry* 2007;164(6):884–91.

84. Bridge JA, Greenhouse JB, Weldon AH, *et al*. Suicide trends among youths aged 10 to 19 years in the United States, 1996–2005. *JAMA* 2008;300(9):1025–6.

85. Bridge JA, Iyengar S, Salary CB, *et al*. Clinical response and risk for reported suicidal ideation and suicide attempts in pediatric antidepressant treatment: a meta-analysis of randomized controlled trials. *JAMA* 2007;297(15):1683–96.

86. National Collaborating Centre for Mental Health. *Depression in children and young people: identification and management in primary, community and secondary care (CG28)*. London: The British Psychological Society; 2005.

CHAPTER 7

ENGAGEMENT

Dennis Ougrin
Saqib Latif

Introduction

As discussed in Chapter 6, the range of effective interventions in adolescent self-harm is increasing. There are two published randomised controlled trials (RCTs) demonstrating the efficacy of both developmental group psychotherapy and multi-systemic therapy on measures of suicidality in adolescents.[1,2]

Despite these advances, poor engagement with follow-up is a major obstacle in providing psychological treatment to adolescents who have self-harmed. Up to 77 per cent of adolescents disengage from outpatient treatment.[3] In a naturalistic follow-up study, half of all the adolescent suicide attempters attended fewer than four follow-up sessions.[4]

Adult literature suggests that disengagement with treatment is one of the strongest predictors of poor outcomes in those presenting to emergency departments.[5] In the adolescent literature there have been studies linking poor engagement with increased suicidality.[6,7] and hopelessness.[8] In addition, there is growing evidence that disengaging coping strategies predict poor psychosocial outcomes and are associated with an increased risk of self-harm.[9] Poor engagement is also seen as a major obstacle to the development and implementation of new effective treatments.[10] Poor engagement seen in clinical practice was one of the key driving forces behind the development of therapeutic assessment.

What factors influence engagement with follow-up?

There are several factors that influence engagement with treatment in young people who have self-harmed. Studies indicate that age and gender,[11] race,[12] low socioeconomic status, severity of psychopathology, substance misuse and antisocial behaviour,[13] poor therapeutic alliance with the therapist and poor appointment scheduling,[14] family and service barriers to treatment participation[15] and parental psychopathology and attitude to treatment,[16,17] all influence engagement with treatment. Young people's experiences in the emergency department (ED) were highlighted as important predictors of further engagement. Time delays between the initial and follow-up appointments,[18] delays in conducting the initial evaluation[12] and the attitudes of ED staff have all been implicated.[19]

On a practical level, the factors associated with poor engagement with treatment could be divided into four groups:[20,21]

1. experiencing stressful events and pragmatic obstacles
2. a poor relationship with the therapist
3. considering treatment to be irrelevant
4. considering treatment to be too demanding.

There are some additional factors associated with improved engagement. They include being treated with medication, having a history of previous contact with mental health services and being reminded about appointments by telephone.[15]

Engagement is a necessary step in therapeutic work although it is not sufficient for clinical improvement. Engagement comprises two related factors: attendance and adherence to treatment. For the purposes of this chapter we will use attendance as a proxy measure for engagement since adherence to the treatment requirements is not reported consistently.[22]

Most controlled studies of psychological therapies for young people who self-harm report the engagement rates achieved and some were specifically designed to improve engagement.[15] However, there are no published systematic reviews reporting the engagement rates achieved in these studies. This chapter comprises such a review and then a pooling together of the results in a meta-analysis.

Method

A literature search was conducted to identify RCTs that compare outpatient specific psychological treatment (SPT) with treatment as usual for adolescents who have self-harmed. OVID, Medline, PsychINFO, EMBASE and PubMed were searched up to the first week of August 2008 using a combination of subject headings and keywords. The reference lists of the retrieved articles were also examined for additional relevant publications and citing articles were also searched. In addition, key investigators in the UK, USA and Australia were contacted to obtain the results of any unpublished studies.

The articles found as a result of the initial search were downloaded into EndNote X2 and duplicates were removed.

Study selection

All RCTs comparing an outpatient SPT and treatment as usual in children or adolescents who had self-harmed recently were included. Self-harm was defined as self-poisoning or self-injury irrespective of the intent.[23] Engagement was defined as attending four or more sessions of a psychotherapeutic intervention. This appeared to be the most consistent cut-off point reported by the reviewed studies. Where this was not clear, the study's corresponding author was contacted to obtain clarification.

The studies with mainly adult samples, studies of pharmacological interventions, studies that included comparisons between outpatient and inpatient treatment, studies not reporting engagement in the format required and studies in which adolescents with self-harm constituted a minority of the study population were excluded.

Data abstraction

For each of the studies, the following information was recorded: details of participants, details of the interventions, participants' flow, intention-to-treat analysis, allocation details and follow-up period (Table 7.1).

Analysis

In the calculation of the risk ratio (risk in this case refers to the risk of not completing four or more sessions of treatment, i.e. not engaging), the outcome of the mean number of sessions attended was used. The subjects in each eligible study were dichotomised into two groups: those attending four or more treatment sessions and those attending fewer than four treatment sessions. The pooled mean effect size was calculated using a computer programme, RevMan (Version 5.0), developed as a support tool in working with the Cochrane review and meta-analyses. Each study was weighted in proportion to its sample size. The variation of study estimates beyond that expected by chance was assessed using Cochrane's test of homogeneity. As there was evidence of significant heterogeneity between the studies, a mean risk ratio was calculated using DerSimonian and Laird's[24] random effect model.

The tau statistic is the standard deviation of the mean number of sessions attended in different studies beyond the variation attributable to the play of chance. We also calculated the I2 statistic, which is another indicator of heterogeneity,[25] in percentages. A value of 0 per cent indicates no observed heterogeneity and larger values show increasing heterogeneity, with 25 per cent as low, 50 per cent as moderate and 75 per cent as high heterogeneity. Results are reported using 95 per cent confidence intervals.

Quality of the studies

Allocation concealment was used as a proxy for the quality of the trials.[26,27] The following quality ratings were applied: (1) adequate concealment (e.g. using opaque sealed envelopes); (2) unclear concealment; (3) inadequate concealment (e.g. using open random numbers tables).

Table 7.1 Selected characteristics of the randomised controlled trials examining the effects of specific psychological treatment versus treatment as usual (TAU) on engagement rates* in adolescents with self-harm

Study	Inclusion criteria	Age	Control	N	Interventions	ITT	Allocation	Follow-up
Spirito et al.[15]	Suicide attempters receiving care in ED or paediatrics ward	12–18	Standard disposition planning	76	Compliance enhancement + standard disposition planning	Subjects completing treatment	Not specified	3 months
Donaldson et al.[28]	Suicide attempters presenting to ED or inpatient unit	12–17	Supportive relationship treatment	39	Skills-based treatment	Subjects starting treatment	Not specified	6 months
Wood et al.[2]	Repeat self harmers referred to an out-patient service	12–16	TAU	63	Developmental group psychotherapy + TAU	Subjects randomised	Concealed	7 months
Harrington et al.[29]	Self poisoning cases referred to mental health teams	<16 (mean 14.5)	TAU	162	Home-based family intervention + TAU	Subjects randomised	Concealed	6 months
King et al.[30]	Suicide attempters, significant suicidality	12–17	TAU	289	Youth-nominated support team – Version 1 + TAU	Subjects randomised	Open	6 months

*Criterion for engagement is attending more than four sessions.
ED, emergency department; TAU, treatment as usual; ITT, intention to treat.

Results

Description of the studies

The original search resulted in the retrieval of 820 articles.

Seven of those described RCTs in children and adolescents with a primary presenting problem of self-harm or suicidality[1,2,15,28–31] and there were five further RCTs in progress or in press.[32–36]

Five of these studies met the inclusion criteria.[2,15,28–30] The selected characteristics of these studies are presented in Table 7.1.

In one of these studies[30] the information on the subjects' engagement was not available in the format required. The remaining four studies were entered into the meta-analysis.

The quality of the studies was variable and randomised allocation concealment was evident in two of the studies.

The engagement reported by the four studies is summarised in Table 7.2.

The reported engagement with an SPT and treatment as usual were compared in the four studies that were included, totalling 340 adolescents. Overall there was no statistically significant difference between the number of subjects not completing four or more sessions of an SPT (29.3 per cent, 79/166) and treatment as usual (47.6 per cent; 51/174), $RR = 0.74$ (95% CI 0.41–1.34) (Figure 7.1).

There was significant heterogeneity between the studies. The small number of studies precluded further subgroup analysis or meta-regression. The study reporting

Table 7.2 Participants' flow and engagement

Study	Eligible	Randomised		Completed follow-up	Attended four or more sessions		Mean total no. of sessions attended		Q
		SPT	TAU		SPT	TAU	SPT	TAU	
Spirito et al.[15]	82	36	40	63	22	23	7.7 (8.4)*	6.4 (5.8)*	2
Donaldson et al.[28]	44	21	18	31	15	16	9.7	9.5	2
Wood et al.[2]	83	32	31	62	23	19	11.5	4	1
Harrington et al.[29]	288	85	77	149	63	28	7.6**	3.6**	1
Kings et al.[30]	697	151	138	236	Not reported	Not reported	Not reported	Not reported	3

*Adjusted for barriers to services; **median.
Q, quality of studies; SPT, specific psychological treatment; TAU, treatment as usual.

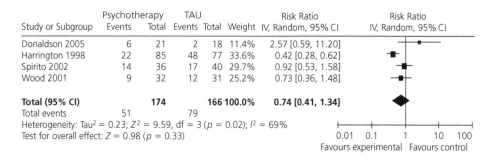

Figure 7.1 Random effects meta-analysis: plot of the studies included in the estimate of the pooled relative risk of the effect of specific psychotherapeutic treatment versus treatment as usual on engagement.

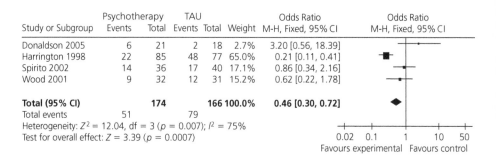

Figure 7.2 Fixed effects meta-analysis: plot of the studies included in the estimate of the pooled odds ratio of the effect of specific psychotherapeutic treatment versus treatment as usual on engagement.

the largest positive effect of a specific (in this case family) psychotherapy on engagement was different from other studies in that the intervention was delivered at home. In that study the proportion of young people attending four or more appointments of routine outpatient care did not differ significantly between the experimental and the control group at 35 per cent versus 39 per cent ($\chi = 0.199$, d.f. = 1, $p = 0.655$) respectively, if the home visits were excluded.

It is of interest that using a different meta-analysis model (fixed effects) could have led to a different conclusion (Figure 7.2). The fixed-effects model is, however, inappropriate in this case as the heterogeneity of the studies is great.

A small number of studies prevented testing for funnel plot asymmetry. Eyeballing the funnel plot did not reveal any small studies with a big effect size favouring interventions over controls, making publication bias unlikely (Figure 7.3).

Discussion

The results of this meta-analysis indicate that there is no evidence of specific psychotherapeutic treatments leading to better engagement than treatment as usual

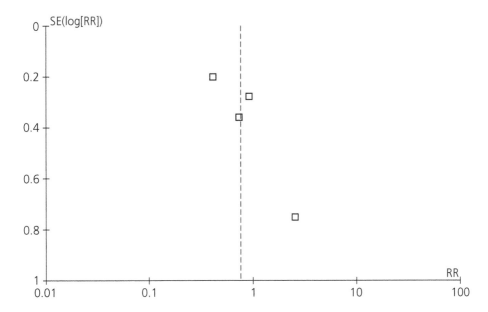

Figure 7.3 Funnel plot of the studies comparing the effect of specific psychotherapeutic treatment versus treatment as usual on engagement. Estimate of the relative risk is plotted against standard error.

in adolescents who have self-harmed. This is of concern given the prevalence of self-harm[37] and the growing evidence base for effective treatment,[2] methods of prevention[38] and an increased understanding of the factors associated with self-harm in general.[39] The absolute difference in engagement rates was not insignificant, however, with 70.7 per cent of SPT cases versus 52.4 per cent of TAU cases completing four or more sessions of treatment. It may be that no statistically significant difference was observed due to insufficient power, thus warranting further research.

The limitations of the studies in this meta-analysis include small sample sizes, uncharacterised treatment as usual (with the exception of Donaldson *et al.*[28]) and non-reporting of the treatment utilisation in non-statutory organisations (with the exception of Harrington *et al.*[29]). A significant proportion of the adolescents presenting with self-harm were excluded or lost to follow up prior to randomisation, further limiting the generalisability of the findings.

The limitations of this meta-analysis are as follows. The small number of studies precluded subgroup analysis. Furthermore, there was significant heterogeneity among the studies. One of the studies was specifically designated to improve adherence[15] whereas the other three had different primary outcome measures. In the study with the largest effect on engagement,[29] a family therapy intervention was delivered by social workers at the subject's home. It is perhaps not surprising that the level of engagement achieved in that study was the greatest. The study with the least favourable effect on engagement compared a challenging, skills training-based therapy with a supportive and manualised treatment delivered by highly trained therapists, i.e. TAU.[28] This TAU was arguably significantly different from the treatment to be expected in ordinary clinical practice.

A second major limitation was the brief follow-up period in all the studies. Although previous literature[17] suggests that the greatest loss of engagement is in the first session of outpatient treatment, it is possible that some adolescents may re-engage at a later date.

Studies included in this meta-analysis have shown better engagement rates overall than some but not all of the previous naturalistic studies.[4,17] It is possible that the engagement with TAU reported by the studies in this meta-analysis is in line with good quality routine clinical practice. However, engagement rates achieved by different services may vary significantly.

For the purposes of this study we used attending four or more sessions as an indicator of engagement. This is necessarily an arbitrary cut-off point, albeit supported by empirical studies.[4] Alternative cut-off points were considered. Attending at least one follow-up session seems a replicable and generally available outcome measure; however, previous studies indicate the importance of dose–response relationships in child psychotherapy[40] which should not be ignored. Equally, the total number of sessions attended provides a good overall picture of engagement with treatment but would generally be prejudicial against those young people who do not attend many appointments because of the resolution of their symptomatology.

Two of the studies were British and two American, each pair using different definitions of self-harm. This difference is unlikely to have influenced the overall conclusion as there is no evidence of differential engagement of young people presenting with suicidal versus non-suicidal self-harm at present.

Is good engagement with follow-up reflected in better outcomes? Although some authors find this to be the case,[8] others question the relationship between engagement and outcomes.[41] It is possible that engagement with SPT leads to better outcomes than engagement with treatment as usual.[6,7,16] There can, however, be little doubt that without good engagement no treatment can be effectively implemented.

SPT is only one factor influencing engagement. Several studies attempted to improve engagement by influencing other factors with variable success. It is unlikely that any one factor in isolation will increase engagement with follow-up appointments.

Summary

Engaging adolescents with psychological treatment is essential, although not sufficient in itself, for improving outcomes. Engagement with outpatient psychotherapy in clinical practice remains poor among adolescents who have self-harmed; however it may be better in clinical trials. There is currently no evidence that outpatient SPT is superior to treatment as usual in improving engagement. Some of the elements that might improve engagement include offering home treatment, tackling service and family barriers to treatment and using the first contact with young people therapeutically. Future research might focus on developing interventions that take into account a range of factors that influence engagement. One of the possible ways forward is therapeutic assessment at the point of first contact with adolescents presenting with self-harm. The results of a therapeutic assessment pilot trial are the subject of Chapter 9.

References

1. Huey SJ, Jr, Henggeler SW, Rowland MD, *et al*. Multisystemic therapy effects on attempted suicide by youths presenting psychiatric emergencies. *J Am Acad Child Adolesc Psychiatry* 2004;43(2):183–90.
2. Wood A, Trainor G, Rothwell J, *et al*. Randomized trial of group therapy for repeated deliberate self-harm in adolescents. *J Am Acad Child Adolesc Psychiatry* 2001;40(11): 1246–53.
3. Trautman PD, Stewart N, Morishima A. Are adolescent suicide attempters noncompliant with outpatient care? *J Am Acad Child Adolesc Psychiatry* 1993;32(1):89–94.
4. Spirito APD, Levy SBA, Kurkjian JPD, *et al*. Adolescent suicide attempts: outcomes at follow-up. *Am J Orthopsychiatry* 1992;62(3):464–8.
5. Cremniter D, Payan C, Meidinger A, *et al*. Predictors of short-term deterioration and compliance in psychiatric emergency patients: A prospective study of 457 patients referred to the emergency room of a general hospital. *Psychiatry Res* 2001;104(1):49–59.
6. Rotheram-Borus MJ, Piacentini J, Cantwell C, *et al*. The 18-month impact of an emergency room intervention for adolescent female suicide attempters. *J Consult Clin Psychol* 2000;68(6):1081–93.
7. Rotherham-Borus MJ, Piacentini J, Van Rossem R, *et al*. Enhancing treatment adherence with a specialized emergency room program for adolescent suicide attempters. *J Am Acad Child Adolesc Psychiatry* 1996;35(5):654–63.
8. Pillay AL, Wassenaar DR. Psychological intervention, spontaneous remission, hopelessness, and psychiatric disturbance in adolescent parasuicides. *Suicide Life Threat Behav* 1995;25(3):386–92.
9. Votta E, Manion I. Suicide, high-risk behaviors, and coping style in homeless adolescent males' adjustment. *J Adolesc Health* 2004;34(3):237–43.
10. Burns J. Clinical management of deliberate self-harm in young people: the need for evidence-based approaches to reduce repetition. *Aust N Z J Psychiatry* 2005;39(3):121–8.
11. Piacentini J, Rotheram-Borus MJ, Gillis JR, *et al*. Demographic predictors of treatment attendance among adolescent suicide attempters. *J Consult Clin Psychol* 1995;63(3): 469–73.
12. Wilder JF, Plutchnik R, Conte HR. Compliance with psychiatric emergency room referrals. *Arch Gen Psychiatry* 1977;34(8):930–3.
13. Pelkonen M, Marttunen M, Laippala P, Lonnqvist J. Factors associated with early dropout from adolescent psychiatric outpatient treatment. *J Am Acad Child Adolesc Psychiatry* 2000;39(3):329–36.
14. Granboulan V, Roudot-Thoraval F, Lemerle S, Alvin P. Predictive factors of post-discharge follow-up care among adolescent suicide attempters. *Acta Psychiatr Scand* 2001;104(1): 31–6.

15. Spirito A, Boergers J, Donaldson D, *et al.* An intervention trial to improve adherence to community treatment by adolescents after a suicide attempt. *J Am Acad Child Adolesc Psychiatry* 2002;**41**(4):435–42.

16. Rotheram-Borus MJ, Piacentini J, Van Rossem R, *et al.* Treatment adherence among Latina female adolescent suicide attempters. *Suicide Life Threat Behav* 1999;**29**(4):319–31.

17. Taylor E, Stansfeld S. Children who poison themselves: II. Prediction of attendance for treatment. *Br J Psychiatry* 1984;**145**:132–5.

18. Clarke CF. Deliberate self poisoning in adolescents. *Arch Dis Child* 1988;**63**(12):1479–83.

19. Rotheram-Borus MJ, Piacentini J, Miller S, *et al.* Toward improving treatment adherence among adolescent suicide attempters. *Clin Child Psychol Psychiatry* 1996;**1**(1):99–108.

20. Kazdin AE, Wassell G. Treatment completion and therapeutic change among children referred for outpatient therapy. *Prof Psychol Res Pr* 1998;**29**(4):332–40.

21. Kazdin AE, Holland L, Crowley M. Family experience of barriers to treatment and premature termination from child therapy. *J Consult Clin Psychol* 1997;**65**(3):453–63.

22. Nock MK, Ferriter C. Parent management of attendance and adherence in child and adolescent therapy: a conceptual and empirical review. *Clin Child Fam Psychol Rev* 2005;**8**(2):149–66.

23. Hawton K, Harriss L, Hall S, *et al.* Deliberate self-harm in Oxford, 1990–2000: a time of change in patient characteristics. *Psychol Med* 2003;**33**(6):987–95.

24. DerSimonian R, Laird N. Meta-analysis in clinical trials. *Control Clin Trials* 1986;**7**(3):177–88.

25. Higgins J, Thompson S, Deeks J, Altman D. Measuring inconsistency in meta-analyses. *BMJ* 2003;**327**(7414):557–60.

26. Schulz KF, Chalmers I, Hayes RJ, Altman DG. Empirical evidence of bias: Dimensions of methodological quality associated with estimates of treatment effects in controlled trials. *JAMA* 1995;**273**(5):408–12.

27. Wood L, Egger M, Gluud LL, *et al.* Empirical evidence of bias in treatment effect estimates in controlled trials with different interventions and outcomes: meta-epidemiological study. *BMJ* 2008;**336**(7644):601–5.

28. Donaldson D, Spirito A, Esposito-Smythers C. Treatment for adolescents following a suicide attempt: results of a pilot trial. *J Am Acad Child Adolesc Psychiatry* 2005;**44**(2):113–20.

29. Harrington R, Kerfoot M, Dyer E, *et al.* Randomized trial of a home-based family intervention for children who have deliberately poisoned themselves. *J Am Acad Child Adolesc Psychiatry* 1998;**37**(5):512–8.

30. King CA, Kramer A, Preuss L, *et al.* Youth-Nominated Support Team for Suicidal Adolescents (Version 1): a randomized controlled trial. *J Consult Clin Psychol* 2006;**74**(1):199–206.

31. Cotgrove AJ, Zirinsky L, Black D, Weston D. Secondary prevention of attempted suicide in adolescence. *J Adolesc* 1995;**18**(5):569–77.

32. Greenhill LL. Treatment of adolescent suicide attempters (TASA) [accessed 30 August 2008] Available from: http://www.clinicaltrials.gov/ct2/show/NCT00080158?term=suicide&age=0&rank=1.

33. Asarnow JR. Effectiveness of a family-based intervention for adolescent suicide attempters (The SAFETY Study) [accessed 30 August 2008] Available from: http://clinicaltrials.gov/ct2/show/NCT00692302.

34. Asarnow JR. Family Intervention for Suicidal Youth: Emergency Care (FISP) [accessed 30 August 2008] Available from: http://clinicaltrials.gov/ct2/show/NCT00558805?term=asarnow&rank=3.

35. Mehlum L. Treatment for adolescents with deliberate self-harm [cited 2008 30 August] Available from: http://www.clinicaltrials.gov/ct2/show/NCT00675129?term=suicide&age =0&rank=2.

36. Chanen AM, Jackson HJ, McCutcheon LK, *et al.* Early intervention for adolescents with borderline personality disorder using cognitive analytic therapy: randomised controlled trial. *Br J Psychiatry* 2008;**193**(6):477–84.

37. Madge N, Hewitt A, Hawton K, *et al.* Deliberate self-harm within an international community sample of young people: Comparative findings from the Child & Adolescent Self-harm in Europe (CASE) Study. *J Child Psychol Psychiatry* 2008;**49**(6):667–77.

38. Aseltine RH, Jr, James A, Schilling EA, *et al.* Evaluating the SOS suicide prevention program: a replication and extension. *BMC Public Health* 2007;**7**:161.

39. Portzky G, De Wilde EJ, van Heeringen K. Deliberate self-harm in young people: differences in prevalence and risk factors between the Netherlands and Belgium. *Eur Child Adolesc Psychiatry* 2008;**17**(3):179–86.

40. Howard KI, Kopta SM, Krause MS, Orlinsky DE. The dose-effect relationship in psychotherapy. *Am Psychol* 1986;**41**(2):159–64.

41. Burns CD, Cortell R, Wagner BM, *et al.* Treatment compliance in adolescents after attempted suicide: a 2-year follow-up study. *J Am Acad Child Adolesc Psychiatry* 2008;**47**(8):948–57.

CHAPTER 8

HOPES AND EXPECTATIONS FROM SELF-HARM ASSESSMENTS: ADOLESCENTS' VERSUS CLINICIANS' VIEWS

Dennis Ougrin
Tobias Zundel

Introduction

In the recent past several qualitative studies have been undertaken to investigate the experiences of those who self-harm. These highlight the difficulties young people have in accessing help.[1] The young people who stopped self-harming indicate that positive interactions with professionals are viewed as an important factor in their recovery.[2] Another study looked into how health services were experienced by people who self-harm,[3] indicating that the service users frequently perceive not being listened to by the professionals. The patients' parents were also the subjects of qualitative studies.[4-6] These revealed parents' feelings of guilt, shame, struggling to understand and perceived lack of support from health professionals.

The outcomes of self-harm assessments are broadly similar irrespective of the profession of the assessor[7] and this was reflected in the National Institute for Health and Clinical Excellence (NICE) guidelines on self-harm,[8] recommending that suitably qualified and supervised professionals provide self-harm assessments. According to the guidelines, all individuals who present with self-harm should have a comprehensive assessment of needs and risk. This assessment should form a part of a therapeutic process to understand and engage the service user. There is a need for further research, including qualitative studies, to advance understanding of the self-harm assessment process, as there is a link between the young people's experience of self-harm assessment and the likelihood of adherence to aftercare.[9,10] As was shown in the previous chapter, the issue of engaging young people is a complex one and a number of factors are at play.

There have been no studies, qualitative or quantitative, focused on the young people's expectations from self-harm assessments. This appears to be a significant gap in knowledge, as understanding and meeting young people's hopes and expectations may be an important step in engaging young people with treatment.

Similarly, there are no studies exploring the hopes and expectations of clinicians who carry out assessments.

The authors of this book conducted a qualitative study to explore the hopes and expectations held by adolescents in relation to being assessed after presenting to health services with self-harm. Assessing clinicians were then interviewed similarly and the findings from the two groups compared. The degree of overlap or difference was considered in terms of how it could impact on the adolescents' subsequent engagement with follow-up.

The study methods

The qualitative in-depth interview study was part of the wider randomised controlled trial of therapeutic assessment, comparing therapeutic assessment versus assessment

---

Box 8.1

Study interview schedule

Question 1

a. Before we start this assessment, I'd like to ask you a slightly unusual question. We might spend the next one hour or so together. After we have finished the assessment, how would you know it was useful?

Clarification prompts

What would tell you that this was not a waste of time?

What are your best hopes from this assessment?

What would be the best thing that could happen as a result of this assessment?

If this assessment was a success, how would you know that it was?

b. Imagine I have a magic wand and anything is possible. If I gave you my magic wand and you could get everything you want from this assessment what would it be?

c. What else? How else would you know this assessment was useful?

d. In what way would the things you have mentioned be good for you?

Question 2.

a. What about slightly longer term? I mean how could this assessment be good for you in the future?

b. What else? How else would you know this assessment was useful?

c. In what way would the things you have mentioned be good for you?

---

as usual (AAU) in young people presenting acutely with self-harm. The first stage in the assessment process explored the young person's expectations of the assessment using a semi-structured interview format (Box 8.1).

The study was undertaken across two London mental health trusts. All services in both trusts routinely follow NICE guidelines for the management of self-harming adolescents, in that a thorough psychosocial assessment is carried out and a follow-up appointment is offered.

Participants

There were two groups of participants in the study. The adolescents presenting with self-harm and the clinicians who carry out self-harm assessments as part of their day-to-day work.

Adolescents

The study population was drawn from a sample of the young people presenting to inner-city psychiatric services for an urgent assessment following an episode of self-harm as defined by Hawton et al.[11]

Table 8.1 Characteristics of the adolescents

Adolescent	Age	Sex	Ethnicity	SH type	Assessment setting	Previous self-harm	Previous MH contact	Main clinical impression
1	15	F	White	OD	ED	No	No	None recorded
2	17	F	White	SI	OPD	Yes	Yes	Substance misuse
3	14	F	White	SI	OPD	Yes	No	None recorded
4	15	F	White	SI	OPD	No	No	Adjustment disorder
5	15	F	White/ Asian	SI	OPD	Yes	No	Depression
6	17	M	Asian	OD	ED	Yes	Yes	Substance misuse
7	16	M	White	SI	OPD	Yes	No	Depression
8	14	F	White/ Asian	SI	OPD	Yes	No	Conduct disorder
9	16	F	Black	SI	OPD	Yes	No	Panic disorder
10	15	F	White	OD	OPD	No	Yes	Agoraphobia

ED, emergency department; MH, mental health; OD, overdose; OPD, outpatient department; SI, self-injury; F, female, M, male; SH, self-harm

After a defined starting date all young people referred for self-harm assessment as part of the authors' routine work were approached for consent to participate in the study. This continued until a total of 10 adolescents had been interviewed (Table 8.1).

Inclusion criteria

Adolescents aged between 12 and 17 years (inclusive) presenting with acute self-harm, either via hospital emergency departments or as urgent family doctor referrals.

Exclusion criteria

Poor English (requiring an interpreter), moderate or severe mental retardation, gross reality distortion due to psychosis or inebriation, an immediate risk of violence or suicide and being admitted to psychiatric inpatient units.

After initial introductions and a routine explanation of the assessment process the authors proceeded to administer the semi-structured interview.

No adolescents refused to participate.

Clinicians

The clinicians were recruited from the control group in the therapeutic assessment for self-harm trial. They had not received any specific training in therapeutic assessment as a result of having been randomised into the AAU arm of this trial. All of the clinicians were experienced mental health workers and their characteristics are described in Table 8.2. The first 10 to respond to invitations for the interview were seen and the semi-structured interview administered.

No clinicians refused to participate.

Table 8.2 Characteristics of the clinicians

Clinician	Age	Sex	Ethnicity	Years of MH experience	Years of Child MH experience	Profession
1	33	M	White	6	4	Doctor
2	42	F	White	6	3	Doctor
3	40	F	White	8	4½	Doctor
4	30	M	White	5	1/2	Doctor
5	30	M	Asian	4	1/2	Doctor
6	28	F	Black	3	1/2	Doctor
7	44	F	Black	12	7	Nurse
8	49	M	White	5	5	Social Worker
9	33	F	Asian	7	6	Psychologist
10	27	M	Asian	2	1/2	Doctor
Mean	36	–	–	6	3	–

MH, mental health; F, female; M, male.

Interviews

The initial interview questions were developed from the original therapeutic assessment manual through discussion with clinicians who routinely carry out this work. Two pilot interviews were conducted prior to commencing the actual study and these were transcribed and subjected to interpretative phenomenological analysis to determine the suitability of the questions.

The duration of each interview was variable but on average lasted approximately 15–20 minutes. A relatively open interview schedule was used, and all the questions were covered in each interview. All interviews were conducted by the authors, and data saturation was reached in each case. With respect to the adolescents interviewed, there had been no previous contact with the authors. Each interview was tape recorded and then transcribed verbatim. At this point the information identifying those interviewed was anonymised.

The initial questions asked were identical for both groups of interviewees.

There were two main questions, each of which was followed by several prompts.

At the end of the interviews with clinicians two further questions were asked. The first question was what the clinicians thought the adolescents would have answered in response to the same questions that they had just been asked. The second question was what the clinicians thought the parents of the adolescents would have answered in response to the initial sequence of questions.

Analysis

The transcripts were analysed sequentially using interpretive phenomenological analysis (IPA).

The aim of IPA is to explore in detail how participants are making sense of their personal and social world and the main currency for an IPA study is the meaning particular experiences, events or states hold for participants.[12]

This approach does not set out to determine facts objectively. It lends itself to the process of establishing and understanding a young person's subjective state prior to a self-harm assessment. The personal preconceptions and individual reflections of researchers are recognised as leading to an interpretive account of the data in this inductive form of analysis.

Triangulation of data, achieved by the authors approaching the same sources and independently coding interviews, reduced the potential for researcher bias.

The process began with reading and re-reading the data several times. The authors then undertook the preliminary coding of the data and worked with independent qualitative researchers to discuss the emerging coding scheme and the coding decisions. All coded data were examined to ensure that the recurrent themes were identified across the dataset. All the themes were included in the results regardless of prevalence and new themes were added as they emerged.

The two authors met repeatedly to check each theme's coded items for consistency, inter-rater agreement and relevance. Finally, the themes were subdivided or grouped as appropriate.

The sequential coding process commenced while the interviews continued to ensure that data saturation was achieved before recruitment terminated.

Once the IPA had been completed for the two sets of data the themes were compared in order to determine similarities and differences.

Results

The separate grouping of the themes for clinicians and for adolescents resulted in a wider range of different themes emerging from the clinicians. There was a degree of overlap between the themes emerging from the clinicians and the themes emerging from the adolescents. The relative importance attributed to these overlapping themes was, however, different between the two groups.

The adolescent group

The following is a summary of the main themes that emerged in this group.

Developing understanding and being listened to

The wish to understand themselves better and feel understood and listened to was raised by 7 of the 10 adolescents. One young person commented that 'just trying to understand would be good' in relation to people understanding her behaviour and not thinking she was 'a freak'.

Most young people were clear that they would value leaving the assessment knowing more about themselves and also their self-harm. They wanted to be able to make sense of what was happening and also understand why: in relation to cutting 'I do feel better afterwards' however 'I'm kind of not really sure why.'

A theme linked to understanding was somehow normalising or feeling more normal about self-harming behaviour. In some cases the adolescents appeared to relate this to being told that there are other young people who also self-harm. One individual responded very clearly when asked how she would know the assessment had been useful: 'Well maybe, if you could make me feel a bit more normal about it.' This idea was also applied to the whole family: 'I'd love it if we could go away for once and be normal as a family'.

Feeling stressed and anxious came up similarly in relation to being understood by others. It was clearly related to the act of self-harm: 'The thing is I cut more when everyone is stressing me out'.

In one case it was clear that at times the person felt totally defined by her behaviour because of other people misunderstanding her core identity: 'Well sometimes it's like all it's about is my cutting, my cutting, it's like I'm this person, I'm the cutter, not me'. This was described as being a particularly difficult problem for other family members, in this case the mother.

Exploring and thinking about change, both in terms of feeling stuck and enhancing motivation for change

Ideas linking self-harm assessment to change were present in half the interviews. This was a complex area. On one hand highlighting the adolescent feeling stuck and powerless, 'It's just ... it's just something that I have to do' 'nothing's gonna change' and being under duress from others 'Everyone keeps telling me I need to change doing what I do.' On the other hand, young people highlighted the importance of enhancing motivation for change, 'Maybe I'd feel I can change things and feel good about it'. The change was seen as important in both themselves 'I'd actually want to change and not give up' and the others 'I wish my mum wasn't around all the time stressing me out'.

Improving interpersonal functioning

This theme arose in every interview. Some young people stated that they would like it 'if everyone would leave me alone' but almost paradoxically then went on to say that they had a real longing to do things together as a close family: 'I'd talk to my mum more'. There was often a clear understanding of how self-harming behaviour would draw in worried and concerned family members and how that is seen as stressful and unnecessary by the adolescents. One adolescent commented on how she might 'push people away sometimes' and how that leaves her feeling alone; another mentioned she gets too engaged and can't say 'no' to others' demands. Regulating relationships was linked to other hopes and expectations discussed here.

Stopping self-harm behaviours and exploring alternatives

Seven out of 10 young people stated they wanted to stop or reduce self-harm and five out of 10 talked specifically about exploring alternative ways of coping. This idea required that the alternatives provide the same kind of relief that was achieved by the self-harm. When prompted some adolescents were able to give examples of other behaviours they might try, like talking to others, listening to music or doing sports, as well as (from the assessors' point of view) less desirable alternatives such as using intoxicating substances and controlling food intake. Most adolescents wanted to have an exploration of the alternatives to self-harm 'to feel I could deal with these [emotions] and you know, do things differently'.

Feeling better and feeling hopeful

Eight out of 10 adolescents stated they wanted to feel better as a result of their assessment: 'I'd be calm ... calmer... and happier'. This theme was linked to the idea of feeling hopeful instead of stuck: 'I'd feel hope that things could be better'. Feeling better was also linked to stopping self-harm: 'I think when I'm happier I wouldn't wanna cut myself as much'. In a number of cases feeling better after the assessment was linked to having been listened to and heard.

The clinicians' group

As already indicated, this group produced a wider range of different themes that could not be grouped together in the process of the IPA. The main themes were:

Engaging the young person

Nine out of 10 clinicians talked about this, but they did not always comment on how it might be achieved: 'I would want to engage the young person really well ...'. Two comments made in response to the question of what would determine if the assessment had gone well were 'that I've been able to engage the young person' and 'if I get the young person to engage in treatment'. It was also stated that the family should be engaged and that this might have an impact on the adolescent attending and making use of their follow-up sessions. The fact that engagement was frequently mentioned suggests an awareness of the unique opportunity provided by an acute assessment.

Carrying out a 'comprehensive assessment'

This was mentioned by 7 out of 10 clinicians. An ideal assessment is when 'you get ... a comprehensive history'. Another clinician said they would know if things had gone well if they had been able to 'make a comprehensive assessment and document everything in detail, to have a detailed assessment'. Several reasons were given for why a comprehensive history is important. These included the idea that it is necessary to help clarify ongoing risk in terms of further self-harm or suicidality: 'The things that would tell me that the assessment was good would be getting all of the risk factors, the risk factors that would predict the future risk. So, risk is obviously the main issue here'. There was also a sense that it was important and reassuring for the clinician to confirm for themselves that on this basis they had done their job well. In addition it was felt to underlie several of the other points including gaining understanding, helping to work with family and establishing pre-existing illness.

A linked theme was that of establishing and addressing any underlying illness with a view to instigating the appropriate treatment as a means of reducing the risk of further self-harm.

Safe disposal and the assessment and management of risk

Eight of the 10 clinicians mentioned one or both of these issues. Safe disposal came up more often than risk itself (7/10 and 4/10 respectively). Risk assessment, therefore, contributed to both the comprehensive assessment and the safe disposal themes. 'I would have done a good risk assessment' was a typical comment and in relation to safe planning this is one of the statements that was made: 'I would want to know that

I came to a safe decision about the young person's future welfare'. In several cases this was perceived as one of the most important goals of the interview. A linked theme was that of harm minimisation. This idea was portrayed by one clinician when asked about the goals of assessment: 'I suppose harm minimisation springs to mind. I suppose we do not have a magic wand or live in an ideal world where you know these things are going to be eradicated. So, something about an ideal goal being minimisation rather than, you know, things escalating or getting more serious or more unhealthy or harmful.'

Improving family relationships and interactions

This was suggested by seven clinicians. One comment about what should be worked on was 'improving the family context, for those who have family difficulties, for them to be better or more healthily shared'. For another clinician it was particularly related to the longer-term impact of the assessment. One clinician thought about working on the 'ability of the family to contribute' towards dealing with the young person's difficulties and another commented, 'They [the family] might become more involved and that could be helpful for the young person'.

Gaining understanding of the young people's behaviour

This was mentioned by 7 of the 10 clinicians. Developing an understanding of the self-harm as well as the context in which it took place was linked to the idea that the young person would feel better. This was related to then looking for alternatives to self-harm or stopping the self-harm completely, the latter seen as a longer-term goal. One clinician was very clear about wanting to be 'able to work with and understand the young person' and another stated with respect to the adolescents: 'Probably, if they get a sense of having been heard and understood, that in itself would have its own therapeutic value and that's something I would keep in mind'.

Predicting the adolescents' hopes and expectations

All clinicians attempted to predict the adolescents' responses to the same set of questions the clinicians had been asked. Many pointed out this was a very good question as it put them in the shoes of their patients. The most frequent responses clustered around the prediction that adolescents probably just wanted to be listened to or heard and that this might help them feel better and more understood.

Discussion

It was possible to obtain codable data from all 20 interviews with those who participated in this study. One adolescent essentially replied 'I don't know' to most questions, stating she did not think her assessment could be useful at all. The 'I don't know' answer was also a common first reply from other young people, but as the interview progressed most young people highlighted a variety of themes. However, it is possible that there may be a significant number of young people who have very little idea about the potential usefulness of the self-harm assessment. This is likely to be more evident if the young people meeting exclusion criteria were interviewed.

The fact that clinicians generated a relatively wider range of themes is perhaps not surprising, but is indicative of the view that adolescents may enter into the assessment process with a more confused and less expectant or purposeful state of mind. Clinicians on the other hand are faced with the challenge of juggling numerous issues that may have to be prioritised differently at different times to achieve the optimal outcome. This was captured by one clinician who said, in relation to documenting extensive histories and completing risk assessment forms, 'There could very easily be a tendency of that bureaucracy to actually sort of kill off getting through to the young person'.

The combination of using a broad definition of self-harm, including consecutive referrals in both acute hospital and outpatient settings improves the generalisability of the findings. However, the findings may not generalise to patient populations beyond inner-city areas. A further threat to generalizability comes from having a small sample size, although data saturation was achieved in all cases. In addition, a broad self-harm definition may obfuscate significant differences between those with and without suicidal intent.[13]

Could addressing young people's hopes and expectations more comprehensively lead to improved engagement with follow-up? This remains to be proven although some initial data suggest it may be the case.[14] There is no conclusive evidence as yet that meeting the young people's expectations of self-harm assessments would improve their engagement with follow-up, let alone long-term psychosocial outcomes. However, there is evidence in other areas that meeting patients' expectations may improve not only engagement but also outcomes.[15]

As was discussed at length in Chapter 7, the process of assessment is only one factor that predicts young people's future engagement with follow-up. There are other factors, including barriers to service access,[16] parental views on the need to attend follow-up,[17] patients' sociodemographic characteristics[18] and stigma, to name but a few.

The differences between the clinicians' and the adolescents' hopes and expectations around self-harm assessment are perhaps predictable. Clinicians are trained to carry out risk assessments and take psychiatric histories. However, being more aware of the young people's views may inform the process of further developing self-harm assessment in such a way that would bear in mind the user's expectations instead of focusing almost exclusively on the clinicians' agenda.

Upon reflection, many clinicians were accurate in predicting the adolescents' hopes and expectations from self-harm assessments, although they predicted a more narrow range of themes than was demonstrated in this study.

This study is the first attempt at investigating young people's hopes and expectations from self-harm assessment. Further studies are needed to explore the relationship between meeting young people's hopes and expectations and their engagement with treatment. It is also important to explore young people's expectations from self-harm assessment in other populations and age groups.

Implications

Clinicians whose work involves the assessment of acute self-harm presentations in adolescents should be aware that their patients may hold different hopes and expectations to their own in relation to the assessment process. More specifically, the clinician is likely to have a wider range of issues in mind, which are likely to have some overlap with the young person, but it may be of particular importance to focus on and address the young people's hopes and expectations in order to facilitate engagement with aftercare.

References

1. Crouch W, Wright J. Deliberate self-harm at an adolescent unit. *Clin Child Psychol Psychiatry* 2004;9:185–204.
2. Sinclair J, Green J. Understanding resolution of deliberate self-harm: qualitative interview study of patients' experiences. *BMJ* 2005;330:1112–4.
3. Arnold L. *Women and self-injury: a survey of 76 women. A report on women's experience of self-injury and their views on service provision*. Bristol: Bristol Crisis Service for Women 1995.
4. Raphael H, Clarke G, Kumar S. Exploring parents' responses to their child's deliberate self-harm. *Health Educ* 2006;106(1):9–20.
5. McDonald G, O'Brien L, Jackson D. Guilt and shame: experiences of parents of self-harming adolescents. *J Child Health Care* 2007;11(4):298–310.
6. Oldershaw A, Richards C, Simic M, Schmidt U. Parents' perspectives on adolescent self-harm: a qualitative study. *Br J Psychiatry* 2008;193:140–4.
7. Weston SN. Comparison of the assessment by doctors and nurses of deliberate self-harm. *Psychiatr Bull* 2003;27:57.
8. National Collaborating Centre for Mental Health. *Self-harm: the short-term physical and psychological management and secondary prevention of self-harm in primary and secondary care*. Clinical Guideline 16. London: Gaskell & British Psychological Society; 2004.
9. Spirito A, Boergers J, Donaldson D, *et al.* An intervention trial to improve adherence to community treatment by adolescents after a suicide attempt. *J Am Acad Child Psychiatry* 2002;41:435–43.
10. Rotheram-Borus MJ, Piacentini J, Van Roosem R, *et al.* Enhancing treatment adherence with a specialized emergency room program for adolescent suicide attempters. *J Consult Clin Psychol* 1996;68:149–66.
11. Hawton K, Hall S, Simkin S, *et al.* Deliberate self-harm in adolescents: a study of characteristics and trends in Oxford, 1990–2000. *J Child Psychol Psychiatry* 2003;44:1191–8.

12. Smith JA. Beyond the divide between cognition and discourse: using interpretative phenomenological analysis in health psychology. *Psychol Health* 1996;**11**:261–71.
13. Nock MK, Kessler RC. Prevalence of and risk factors for suicide attempts versus suicide gestures: analysis of the National Comorbidity Survey. *J Abnorm Psychol* 2006;**115**:616–23.
14. Ougrin D, Ng A, Low J. Therapeutic assessment based on cognitive-analytic therapy for young people presenting with self-harm: pilot study. *Psychiatr Bull* 2008;**32**:423–6.
15. Joe GW, Simpson DD, Dansereau DF, *et al.* Relationship between counselling rapport and drug abuse treatment outcomes. *Psychiatr Serv* 2001;**52**:1223–9.
16. Kazdin AE, Bass D, Ayers WA, Rodgers A. Empirical and clinical focus of child and adolescent psychotherapy research. *J Consult Clin Psychol* 1990;**5**:729–40.
17. Nock MK, Photos V. Parent motivation to participate in treatment: Assessment and prediction of subsequent participation. *J Child Fam Stud* 2006;**15**:345–58.
18. Cremniter D, Payan C, Meidinger A, *et al.* Predictors of short-term deterioration and compliance in psychiatric emergency patients: a prospective study of 457 patients referred to the emergency room of a general hospital. *Psychiatry Res* 2001;**104**:49–59.

CHAPTER 9

TESTING THERAPEUTIC ASSESSMENT IN REAL LIFE

Dennis Ougrin

Introduction

In the previous chapters it was shown that self-harm is a serious and prevalent condition affecting many adolescents. There are efficient and probably effective interventions for adolescent self-harm, but overall poor engagement may be a significant impediment to their delivery. Finally, there was a discussion around the possible reasons why this poor engagement might be so difficult to tackle.

This chapter describes the first pilot study of therapeutic assessment (TA). It does not dwell on the model itself as this is fully described in the latter part of this book. The chapter outlines the way in which TA was tested in an inner-London outpatient and emergency hospital setting.

Hypothesis

It was hypothesised that using TA as an add-on to assessment as usual would improve attendance at the first follow-up appointment and engagement with treatment over a period of 17 weeks, compared with routine assessment as usual.

Participants

Adolescents aged 12–18 who had harmed themselves and were receiving medical care in either the emergency department (ED) or the paediatric wards of two inner-London hospitals, or who were referred by a family doctor to a tertiary community child psychiatry team for an urgent outpatient department (OPD) appointment following an act of self-harm, were eligible for the project. The exclusion criteria included gross reality distortion (for example due to psychotic illness or intoxication), known history of moderate or more severe mental retardation, lack of fluent English, severe risk of violence and the need for inpatient psychiatric treatment. Adherence to follow-up was ascertained for all the young people who required outpatient treatment. An act of self-harm was defined as any self-injury, regardless of the apparent intent or lethality, which was reported as an attempt to harm or kill oneself.[1]

Therapist training and matching

Seven front-line clinicians who were interested in undertaking training in TA and who had no previous training in cognitive analytic therapy (CAT) were chosen. These clinicians had five 2-hour training sessions in TA. The clinicians were then divided into two groups matched on the following variables: mental health experience, age, sex and ethnicity.

Four out of seven continued to assess the adolescents using assessment as usual (AAU) and three clinicians implemented TA in addition to a standard evaluation in all of the eligible adolescents referred to them for assessment.

Procedure

Eligible participants were approached about being in the project after they had been medically stabilised. Adolescents were assessed using the International Classification of Diseases, tenth revision (ICD-10)[2] criteria. Participants in the TA group also completed two questionnaires assessing their level of distress prior to the presentation (very distressed, distressed, not distressed) and their satisfaction with the assessment (satisfied, fairly satisfied, unsatisfied).

After the relevant consent/assent agreements were signed the young people were assessed using either AAU or TA. This procedure was approved by the South London and Maudsley NHS Mental Health Trust and the Institute of Psychiatry's Research Ethics Committee.

Participant flow

Over a period of 5 months, the seven therapists received a total of 38 referrals of young people for self-harm assessment. Nineteen cases (14 female, 5 male) were referred to the three therapists who were required to perform TA and 19 (16 female, 5 male) to the four therapists who continued AAU. Thirty-one of the referred young people met inclusion criteria and agreed to participate. One young person was lost to follow-up but was nonetheless included in the intention-to-treat analysis. All of the therapists participated in regular self-harm on-call duties and carried out urgent assessments in Child and Adolescent Mental Health Services (CAMHS). Cases and controls were ascertained by asking the therapists to keep a log of their referrals and cross-checking with the hospital's electronic patient records (EPRs) as well as the community teams' EPRs.

Standard assessment and follow-up planning (assessment as usual)

Patients' discharge and follow-up was based on the judgement of the clinicians who conducted the evaluation. Three of the eligible adolescents were admitted to an inpatient psychiatric facility and were not included in the final analysis. All of those young people discharged home received a follow-up appointment within seven working days in accordance with National Institute for Health and Clinical Excellence (NICE) guidelines.[1] The assessment letter was sent to the relevant community team and a copy was sent to the family in accordance with the copying letters to patients' policy of the Mental Health Trust.

Fidelity to standard psychosocial assessment (AAU)

This was measured by two independent raters comparing the assessment letters with the gold-standard assessment criteria derived from the NICE guidelines[1] (Table 9.1)

A total of six (30 per cent) of the available therapists' evaluations were rated to determine whether they were adequately completed. Adherence to these 17 points

Table 9.1 Components of the psychosocial assessment to be covered as recommended by the National Institute for Clinical Excellence.

Component	Described (+, −, NA)
Interview alone and with carer if present	
Demographic characteristics	
Characteristics of the act	
Suicidal intent	
Motivation for the act	
Life events	
Substance misuse	
Family composition	
Psychiatric history	
Previous self-harm	
Physical health	
Social situation	
School performance	
Criminality/violence	
Mental state	
Hopelessness	
Need for child protection	

NA, not available.

averaged 71 per cent (minimum 59 per cent, maximum 82 per cent, SD 9.6 per cent). Agreement between the raters on six cases averaged 92 per cent (minimum 76 per cent, maximum 100 per cent, SD 9.8 per cent).

Therapeutic assessment

Following a standard psychosocial history a 30-minute therapeutic session was conducted by the therapist. The major components of the TA were as follows:

1. standard psychosocial history and risk assessment
2. 10-minute break
3. joint construction of a diagram based on the CAT paradigm. The diagram consisted of three elements: identifying reciprocal roles, identifying the 'core pain' and identifying the maladaptive procedures
4. identifying the target problem
5. considering the motivation for change and using motivational interviewing if motivation appeared low
6. searching for potential 'exits' i.e. ways of breaking the vicious cycles identified. This was facilitated by the following techniques
   - examining the influence and control of the target problem on the young person's self, family and social network
   - looking for any exits tried in the past and exploring the present options
   - using future-oriented reflexive questioning
   - using problem-solving techniques
   - exploring alternative views of 'core pain'
   - behavioural techniques, including relaxation.
7. summarising the issues discussed in an understanding letter.

The aims of TA were fourfold:

1. develop a joint understanding of the young person's difficulties
2. enhance motivation for change
3. instil hope
4. explore possible alternatives to self-harm.

Therapeutic assessment was manualised, although the assessing professionals used their clinical judgement when deciding on the best approach to 'exits'. All professionals received five 1-hour group supervision sessions at monthly intervals throughout the duration of the trial.

We used an EPR system to monitor the adherence to the outpatient appointments and contacted the allocated case manager to ascertain the adherence figures.

Fidelity to therapeutic assessment

To ensure fidelity to TA, 30 per cent of the clinicians' letters were rated by an independent rater on seven points that are required to be covered in TA (Table 9.2).

Table 9.2 Components of the therapeutic assessment Understanding Letter

Component	Described (+, –, NA)
Acknowledgement of cooperation	
Preliminary description of reciprocal roles	
Preliminary description of core pain	
Preliminary description of procedural loop	
At least one exit discussed	
Invitation for further work	
Invitation to attend/details of the next follow-up	

NA, not available.

Adherence averaged 87 per cent and ranged from 49 per cent to 94 per cent (SD 18 per cent). Agreement between the raters averaged 97 per cent.

In addition, five audiotaped TA sessions were reviewed by a panel of investigators to confirm adherence to the manual.

Fidelity to basic assessment in the therapeutic assessment group

We also assessed the quality of the basic psychosocial assessment in the TA group. A total of six (30 per cent) of the available therapists' evaluations were rated to determine whether they were adequately completed. An independent rater rated the clinicians' adherence to 17 points that the NICE collaborators deemed as being important to cover in a standard clinical evaluation (Table 9.1), such as assessment of ongoing suicidality. Adherence to these 17 points averaged 89 per cent (minimum 82 per cent, maximum 94 per cent, SD 5.9 per cent). Agreement between the raters on six cases averaged 95 per cent (minimum 88 per cent, maximum 100 per cent, SD 4.5 per cent).

Therapists

Seven mental health professionals were trained in TA. The therapists included two White men and one Indian man, two White women, one Black woman and one Indian woman. Five of the therapists were psychiatric trainees (senior house officers and specialist registrars); there was one nurse and one clinical psychologist. The therapists were matched for mental health experience age, sex and ethnicity (Table 9.3).

Baseline assessment measures

This pilot study was designed to be as close to routine clinical practice as possible. Assessment as usual included no extra measures beyond those recorded as a matter

Table 9.3 Therapists' characteristics

Characteristic	AAU	TA
Male : Female	2:2	1:2
Average age	31. 5	30.7
Psychiatric experience (years)	4.1	4.0
White: non-White	2:2	2:1
British: non-British	3:1	2:1

AAU, assessment as usual; TA, therapeutic assessment

of routine practice. The young people in the TA group filled out two three-point Likert scale questionnaires rating their level of distress in the past 2 weeks as well as their appraisal of how helpful TA had been.

Sociodemographic variables such as age, gender, race and the family's socioeconomic status were recorded. Characteristics of self-harm were also recorded.

Clinical impression based on ICD-10 diagnostic criteria

Clinical impressions were based on the ICD-10. Clinical assessment focused on the conditions frequently found in adolescents who self-harm – depression, anxiety, disruptive behavioural disorders, psychosis, eating disorders and substance misuse. This process resulted in the recording of a clinical impression but did not involve any extra forms or interviews beyond routine clinical practice.

Follow-up

All patients were followed up for an average of 17 weeks after the emergency presentation. The type of treatment offered and the length of treatment were not influenced by the researchers in any way. However, the person responsible for the follow-up (case manager) received a letter detailing the assessment process. If TA was used, a standard psychosocial assessment letter and the 'understanding letter' were sent to the case manager. If AAU was used, a standard psychosocial letter was sent to the case manager. We ascertained the adherence to the follow-up arrangements using the electronic patient records database and by contacting the relevant case manager directly.

The following indexes of the engagement with follow-up were measured:

1. Attendance at the first (7-day) follow-up appointment.
2. Engagement with services. This, following a period of consultation with clinicians, was operationalised as attending 50 per cent or more of the appointments offered (excluding those cancelled by either the patient or the therapist).

Statistical analysis

All patients in each group were compared on baseline and follow up measures, using t-tests for continuous variables and χ^2 tests for dichotomous variables.

Results

Preliminary analyses

Baseline characteristics

There were no significant differences between the two groups on most of the demographic and clinical baseline characteristics studied (Table 9.4), apart from the assessment setting. Assessments were more likely to have occurred in the OPD than in the ED in the TA group.

Attitudes of young people towards therapeutic assessment

Of the 16 young people who had TA, eight (50 per cent) considered TA to have been helpful, six (38 per cent) fairly helpful, one (6 per cent) unhelpful and data were missing in one (6 per cent) case. Young people who rated their experience as helpful were no more likely to attend the first follow-up ($\chi^2 = 1.50$, non-significant (ns)) or to engage with treatment ($\chi^2 = 0.19$, ns) than others.

Assessment of distress

Of the 16 young people who had TA, 11 (69 per cent) described themselves as 'very distressed' in the past 2 weeks before the assessment, three (19 per cent) as fairly distressed and two (12 per cent) as not distressed. Young people who indicated they were 'very distressed' were no more likely to attend the first follow-up appointment ($\chi^2 = 0.1$, ns) or to engage with treatment ($\chi^2 = 1.25$, ns) than others.

Effects of therapeutic assessment on the adherence to follow-up

Assessment and follow-up in the therapeutic assessment group

There were 19 referrals made. One young person was excluded due to the therapist having a clinical impression of psychotic illness. Sixteen young people were offered TA and all agreed to participate, with the guardian's consent. Two young people who were not offered TA presented together (both with self-harm) and the assessing therapist did not offer TA because of a perceived shortage of time. One of the young people was nonetheless subsequently offered a follow-up appointment and the other was admitted to an inpatient facility (and therefore excluded). In total, 16 young people were offered outpatient follow-up, two were admitted to an inpatient facility and one young person was considered in no need of follow-up because of the minor nature of

Table 9.4 Baseline characteristics

Characteristic	TA (n = 19)	AAU (n = 19)	χ^2	p
Mean age	15	14.7	$t = 2.0$	NS
SD	1.25	1.89		
Female (%)	16 (84)	14 (73)	0.63	NS
Ethnicity				
White British	13 (68)	13 (68)	0.00	NS
Black British	5 (28)	4 (21)	0.15	NS
Other	1 (5)	2 (11)	0.36	NS
Method				
Overdose	10 (52)	13 (68)	0.99	NS
Self-injury	7 (37)	5 (28)	0.49	NS
Other	2 (11)	1 (5)	0.36	NS
Assessment setting				
Outpatient department	9 (47)	3 (17)	4.38	p<0.05
Emergency department	10 (52)	16 (83)		
Previous self-harm	13 (68)	9 (47)	1.72	NS
Previous contact with mental health services	5 (28)	4 (21)	0.15	NS
Family SES				
Professional	1 (5)	2 (11)	0.36	NS
Skilled	12 (67)	11 (61)	0.08	NS
Unskilled	3 (17)	3 (17)	0.00	NS
Data missing	2 (11)	2 (11)	0.00	NS
Inpatient admission*	2 (11)	3 (17)	0.23	NS
Clinical impression				
Adjustment disorder	6 (32)	9 (47)	0.99	NS
Depression	4 (11)	2 (11)	0.79	NS
No mental illness	4 (21)	6 (32)	0.54	NS
Other	5 (28)	2 (11)	1.58	NS
On psychotropic medication**	2 (11)	2 (11)	0.00	NS

*Psychiatric hospitalisation; **at the time of assessment.
NS, not significant; SO, standard deviation; SES, socioeconomic status.

the self-harm and there being no evidence of mental illness. All of the referrals made were traceable. Twelve (75 per cent) of the young people attended the first follow-up appointment. Of the original 16 young people who were referred for the outpatient treatment, 13 were considered in need of ongoing treatment. Of those, eight (62 per cent) engaged with services as operationalised by the investigators.

Assessment and follow-up in the assessment-as-usual group

In the AAU group, there were also 19 referrals. All were offered AAU. One young person did not wait for the assessment. She, nonetheless, was subsequently offered a follow-up appointment. An outpatient follow-up appointment was offered in 15 cases (one young person was deemed to be in no need of psychiatric follow-up and three young people were admitted to inpatient psychiatric units). One young person was lost to follow-up, as the team responsible for the follow-up did not receive the referral. Six (40 per cent) young people attended the first appointment. Ten young people were deemed in need of on-going treatment and three (30 per cent) of those engaged with the services as operationalised by the authors.

The survival curves in both groups are detailed in Figure 9.1.

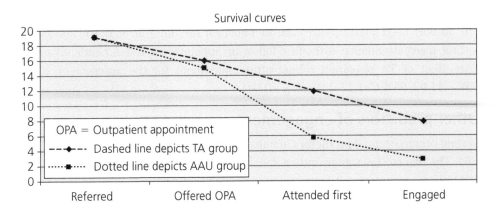

Figure 9.1 Engagement with outpatient follow-up after assessment: therapeutic assessment versus assessment as usual. OPA, outpatient appointment. Dashed line, therapeutic assessment group; dotted line, assessment as usual group.

There were no significant differences between the two groups on the baseline characteristics studied (Table 9.4) apart from the assessment setting. This was more likely to have occurred at a tertiary CAMHS than in the ED in the TA group and reflected the relevant clinicians' work setting.

A direct comparison of the attendance at the first follow-up appointment revealed a statistically significant difference between TA and AAU: 75 per cent (12 out of 16) versus 40 per cent (6 out of 15) (χ^2 [1, N = 31] = 3.89, p <0.05). There was also a statistically significant difference between the two groups on subsequent engagement with services: 62 per cent (8 out of 13) versus 30 per cent (3 out of 10) (χ^2 [1, N = 23] = 4.49, p < 0.05).

Table 9.5 Predictors of attendance at the first follow-up appointment and engagement with follow-up

Factor	First follow-up (significance)	Engagement (significance)
Female sex	1.17 (NS)	4.74 ($p<0.05$)
White British ethnicity	1.98 (NS)	2.22 (NS)
Previous contact	1.99 (NS)	0.6 (NS)
Previous self-harm	2.42 (NS)	5.79 ($p<0.05$)
High social class	0.17 (NS)	0.98 (NS)
Same-sex assessor	0.02 (NS)	0.63 (NS)
Same-ethnicity assessor	0.04 (NS)	0.65 (NS)
Follow-up by assessor	1.17 (NS)	4.28 ($p<0.05$)

NS, not significant.

Effect of intervention accounting for potential confounders

The authors used logistic regression to adjust for the differences in the assessment setting, using attendance at the first follow-up appointment as a dependent variable. The effect of TA remained robust after adjustment for the assessment setting (OR = 11.92, 95% CI 1.27–112.22, $p <0.04$).

Other predictors of engagement

Several other potential predictors of subsequent engagement were measured (Table 9.5). The two factors significantly associated with adherence to follow-up (male sex and history of previous self-harm) were only significant when considering engagement with treatment and did not significantly predict the attendance at the first (7-day) follow-up appointment.

Discussion

This study focused on the improvement of adherence to community follow-up, which has been identified as one of the principal obstacles in delivering psychological therapy to adolescents presenting with self-harm. The results show a statistically significant increase in the rate of attendance at the first community follow-up after TA versus AAU. This study also showed that attending the first follow-up is linked to engagement with treatment in the medium term. Compared with other studies in this field,[3–5] this study shows a more robust improvement in adherence to follow-up, although it is weaker methodologically. Several issues need to be considered as possible explanations for these findings.

First, Spirito et al.[4] showed that one of the strongest predictors of poor adherence to treatment in the USA was 'barriers to services'. These are conventionally divided into family and service barriers.[6] It is of interest that many of the service barriers described (e.g. problems with insurance coverage) do not apply in the UK in the same way. NICE guidelines[1] requiring 7-day follow-up for all young people presenting with self-harm have virtually eliminated a further three potential barriers (being placed on a waiting list, delays in getting appointments or a service reporting no further need for treatment). One of the factors potentially contributing to service barriers in the UK is that the person conducting the initial self-harm assessment is not (with some exceptions) expected to provide follow-up. Interestingly, data from this study support the notion that the same therapist providing follow-up may lead to better engagement in the medium term, although no significant difference for the first (7-day) follow-up attendance was shown. This is consistent with other reported findings.[7]

Owing to the pragmatic design of the study the impact of family barriers on adherence to follow-up was not assessed (e.g. language barriers could not have been assessed, as non-fluent English was an exclusion criterion). The data do not support the notion that young people from higher socioeconomic backgrounds are more likely to engage, and the young people's attitude towards TA did not predict their adherence either.

Beyond the family barriers, it is worth considering wider cultural variables, including the issues of stigma, peer pressure and the attitudes to self-harm in the young people's environment. This was not specifically addressed in the study but has been tackled by other researchers.[8,9]

Second, the method used (TA) is an eclectic tool with an emphasis on clinical judgement and the recognition of a wide variety of needs that young people presenting with self-harm have. The authors propose that using a single therapeutic modality (e.g. a problem-solving intervention, psychoeducation or family therapy) in the assessment of young people presenting with self-harm is unlikely to engage all such young people, and a variety of therapeutic tools may need to be used to achieve the best result. This of course has implications for training and evaluation, but is closer to real-life ED work.

The controversial nature of the relationship between engagement with treatment and outcomes has been discussed above. The following studies are also pertinent to adolescents with emergency presentations of self-harm. Stewart et al.[10] showed an association between poor adherence and suicide re-attempts following an emergency psychiatric presentation. Trautman and Shaffer[11] demonstrated an association between non-attendance and both persistent suicidality and severity of psychopathology.

However, although an association between the outcome and adherence to follow-up has been established, causality has not been demonstrated.

Limitations

Several limitations should be considered in this study. First, the design of the study was quasi-experimental and therefore all of the limitations of non-randomised studies apply. Perhaps some of the most important factors that have not been controlled for are the therapists' variables. We have attempted to match the therapists as much as possible on factors such as age, experience, sex and ethnicity, but there may have been other characteristics like therapeutic style and interpersonal skills that are much more difficult to measure.

Could other factors have affected the outcomes of the study? It is possible that certain patients' characteristics may have influenced the adherence to follow-up. We did not undertake extensive baseline assessment measures and it is therefore impossible to have a precise estimate of the influence of the severity of psychopathology on the outcome. This was done for three reasons. First, the study gained by keeping the trial conditions as close to real life as possible. Second, previous studies commented on the difficulties of administering comprehensive assessment tools in the ED and, third, these studies also highlighted the limited predictive value of these measures with respect to the outcome.[4]

Our results could have been less robust if the young people admitted to inpatient psychiatric facilities were included in the analysis. Inpatient admission in adolescents presenting with self-harm is not common in the UK, but this highlights limitations in the generalisablity of the findings to other settings. Similar US studies indicate a significantly higher proportion of young people presenting with self-harm being admitted to inpatient facilities as well as being prescribed psychotropic medication.[3,4] Both these factors appear to significantly increase the adherence to follow-up.

Finally, the NICE guidelines stipulate that all under-16-year-olds presenting with self-harm are to be admitted overnight to a paediatric ward. This creates favourable conditions for TA in the UK. Were young people likely to be assessed in the immediate aftermath of self-harm, TA might be problematic because of the level of distress and time considerations.

Summary

It is generally recognised that attrition rates are a particular problem in the development of effective interventions in adolescents presenting with self-harm. This chapter presented the data from the first evaluation of TA in a trial. Bearing in mind the limitations, TA showed the potential to improve engagement in follow-up treatment after an urgent presentation with self-harm. The study showed that it is feasible to establish a training programme in TA with inbuilt evaluation and supervision. It also showed few impediments to a wider application of TA in both the ED setting and in the OPD. It may be important to evaluate this method in non-urgent cases of self-harm and perhaps in other patient groups. It remains to be seen if the increased adherence to follow-up holds in a more rigorous random allocation study. More importantly, it will be essential to evaluate a range of psychosocial outcomes in the young people assessed with TA over a longer period of time.

This study adds to the growing evidence that a therapeutic session incorporated into the process of assessing young people who present with self-harm may result in greater adherence to outpatient follow-up.

References

1. National Collaborating Centre for Mental Health. *Self-harm: the short-term physical and psychological management and secondary prevention of self-harm in primary and secondary care*. Clinical Guideline 16. London: Gaskell & British Psychological Society; 2004.
2. World Health Organization. *International classification of diseases*, tenth revision. Geneva: WHO, 1992.
3. Rotherham-Borus MJ, Piacentini J, Van Rossem R, Graae F, *et al*. Enhancing treatment adherence with a specialized emergency room program for adolescent suicide attempters. *J Am Acad Child Adolesc Psychiatry* 1996;**355**:654–63.
4. Spirito A, Boergers J, Donaldson D, Bishop D, Lewander W. An intervention trial to improve adherence to community treatment by adolescents after a suicide attempt. *J Am Acad Child Adolesc Psychiatry* 2002;**414**:435–42.
5. Zimmerman JK, Asnis GM, Schwartz BJ. Enhancing outpatient treatment compliance: A multifamily psychoeducational intake group. In: Zimmerman JK, Asnis GM, editors. *Treatment approaches with suicidal adolescents*. Oxford, UK: John Wiley & Sons; 1995: pp. 106–34.
6. Kazdin AE, Wassell G. Barriers to treatment participation and therapeutic change among children referred for conduct disorder. *J Clin Child Psychol* 1999;**282**:160–72.
7. Torhorst A, Moller HJ, Burk F, Kurz A, Wachtler C, Lauter H. The psychiatric management of parasuicide patients: a controlled clinical study comparing different strategies of outpatient treatment. *Crisis* 1987;**81**:53–61.
8. Huey SJ, Jr, Henggeler SW, Rowland MD, Halliday-Boykins CA, Cunningham PB, Pickrel SG, *et al*. Multisystemic therapy effects on attempted suicide by youths presenting psychiatric emergencies. *J Am Acad Child Adolesc Psychiatry* 2004;**432**:183–90.
9. King CA, Kramer A, Preuss L, *et al*. Youth-Nominated Support Team for Suicidal Adolescents (Version 1): a randomized controlled trial. *J Consult Clin Psychol* 2006;**741**:199–206.
10. Stewart SE, Manion IG, Davidson S, Cloutier P. Suicidal children and adolescents with first emergency room presentations: predictors of six-month outcome. *J Am Acad Child Adolesc Psychiatry* 2001;**405**:580–7.
11. Trautman PD, Shaffer D. Pediatric management of suicidal behavior. *Pediatr Ann* 1989;**182**:134.

CHAPTER 10

THERAPEUTIC ASSESSMENT OVERVIEW

Dennis Ougrin

Introduction

Therapeutic assessment (TA) is a brief therapeutic intervention that forms an organic part of the psychosocial assessment following an act of self-harm. It is aimed at achieving the following goals:

- to help the young person understand their difficulties
- to instil hope and set targets
- to explore and enhance motivation
- to explore possible alternatives to self-harm.

These factors relate to what emerged from the qualitative research, discussed in Chapter 8, that looked into the hopes and expectations held by adolescents in relation to the self-harm assessment. Before being assessed, the young people were asked a number of questions, including: 'How would you know that this assessment had been useful?' Interestingly, most assessors agreed that these objectives are indeed important and this is how a method of rating TA was introduced. A practical extension of these goals is to engage the young person in follow-up after an episode of self-harm.

The next three diagrams represent the TA process (Figures 10.1–10.3).

If everything is clear after reviewing these diagrams, congratulations – you are ready to use TA. Alternatively, please have a cup of coffee and continue reading – you are more than halfway through the book already!

We will now briefly revisit the four main targets of TA.

Developing a joint understanding of the young person's difficulties

Therapeutic assessment uses the cognitive analytic therapy (CAT) paradigm to achieve this goal. A detailed algorithm of constructing CAT diagrams is presented in Chapter 12. Here we will discuss the basic premises of CAT.

Assessment Manual

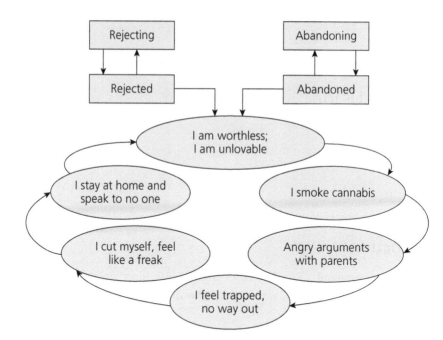

Figure 10.1 Therapeutic assessment diagram.

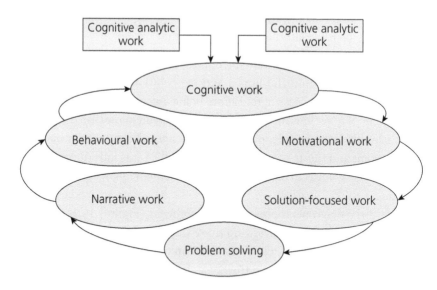

Figure 10.2 Therapeutic assessment diagram with targets.

Cognitive analytic therapy is a brief focal therapy based on the principles of cognitive–behavioural therapy, psychodynamic psychotherapy and cognitive psychology. It was developed by Anthony Ryle for the National Health Service (NHS). This work was informed by ideas derived from object relations theory and Vygotskian ideas on activity and development.

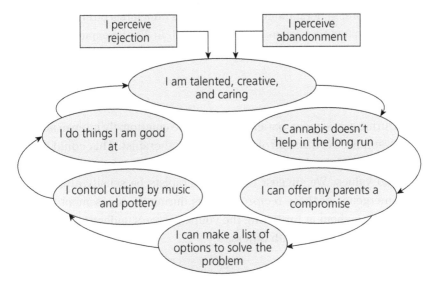

Figure 10.3 Therapeutic assessment diagram with exits.

Cognitive analytic therapy offers a pragmatic problem-solving focus that is based on the understanding of problematic relationship patterns called reciprocal roles (please refer to Chapter 12 for an in-depth discussion of reciprocal roles). Although the original CAT studies have been done with patients suffering from personality disorders and emerging borderline personality disorder in particular, it soon became clear that CAT ideas could be applied to a range of conditions.[1]

The CAT understanding of self-harm is based on an assumption that only a limited range of problematic reciprocal roles are consciously or unconsciously adopted. Moreover, the reciprocal roles tend to switch frequently and wildly and are subject to limited self-reflection and self-control. Human personality is understood as being formed by internalising reciprocal role relationships that emerge during early development. On the one hand, reciprocal role switches lead to the formation of 'core pain' – central negative ideas and feelings about the self. On the other hand, they give rise to problematic patterns of behaviour or *procedural sequences* or *procedures*. Core pain is described as both a reason for and a result of the enactment of the problematic procedures.

In TA the authors propose a modified version of these procedure descriptions. They usually take a circular form and are designed in such a way that each point in the diagram could provide a target for future interventions.

The procedures of a given patient can be summarised in a sequential diagram. The diagram and the link between past experiences and present problems are described in an 'understanding letter'. All elements of the diagram are constructed with the patient's participation and using their descriptions.

Assessment Manual

The procedural understanding of the patient's difficulties often suggests '*exits*', i.e. ways of breaking the vicious cycles identified. In TA the exploration of exits is of paramount importance and is informed by a range of evidence-based approaches.

Note

During assessment, patients may induce emotionally intense and dysphoric reciprocal-role states in the therapist. This could be partly explained by the therapist's own life experiences, beliefs and values. We suggest that the therapists be sensitive to the emergence of these reciprocal roles during the assessment and may use them in furthering the young person's understanding of how they interact with others.

2 Exploring and enhancing motivation for change

This is done via a step-by-step exploration of the pros and cons of a problematic behaviour, assessing different components of motivation, eliciting change talk, enhancing motivation and preparing a change plan using principles of motivational interviewing. Successful motivational work will help the young person clarify or even establish goals and targets and is a crucial element in the improvement of adherence to follow-up. Exploring and enhancing motivation to change could be an exit in its own right or it could precede exploration of other exits.

Instilling hope

The main purpose of this is to address hopelessness and hopefulness in relation to the TA. This part is aimed at supporting the young person's expectations and hopes and noting evidence-based positive predictive factors. It also links the young person's views and expectations with those of the family members and the wider social network. Setting a clear target is seen as part of the process.

Explore possible 'exits': ways to break the vicious cycles

The following techniques could be used to explore the possible exits:

- examining the influence and control of the target problem on the young person's self, family and social network and externalising the problem;
- looking for exits that were tried in the past and exploring those times when the problem was least powerful;

- using future-oriented reflexive questioning, based on the idea that the young person has a good reason for their behaviour but also has power and resources to change it;
- using problem-solving to explore a range of possible solutions;
- exploring alternative views of 'core pain' and challenging self-defeating thoughts;
- behavioural techniques likely to disrupt the vicious cycles, including relaxation and activity scheduling.

It is possible that in the future many more techniques may be used in TA. Therapeutic assessment is a 'toolbox', and any evidence-based technique that could help break the vicious cycles identified may, and perhaps should, be incorporated. The idea is that a therapist will be confident in using several tools of TA, just like a good artist could use several techniques to convey their way of seeing the world. Granted, one of those techniques may be the artist's favourite, but restricting themselves to this could be a disservice to both the artist and the audience.

Imagine that Leonardo continued to use only pen and ink for the rest of his paintings.

References

1. Ryle A, Kerr I. *Introduction to cognitive analytic therapy: principles and practice.* New York: Wiley, 2002.

CHAPTER 11

HISTORY TAKING

Tobias Zundel

Full psychiatric history and mental state

The following is a guide to taking a psychiatric history in the context of a self-harm presentation. Thorough risk assessment and management is usually the cornerstone of the assessment from a health service's point of view. Young people however tend to view this as being a less important component of the assessment. What they are more likely to expect is to be understood, to be respected and to get something useful out of the assessment. Taking a psychosocial history is therefore a skilful balance between the needs of the young person and your own needs as a representative of a health service. These needs are not mutually exclusive and could be complementary. You may try to develop understanding, instil hope, enhance motivation and explore alternatives to self-harm in return for the young person sharing their intimate information with you.

Introduction

For the purposes of therapeutic assessment (TA) the aim of the basic psychosocial history is to generate the information required to be able to construct a diagram depicting the young person's difficulties. It is suggested that clinicians spend 30–60 minutes completing a full history and mental state examination.

Taking a comprehensive psychosocial history and mental state examination is one of the fundamental skills learned early on in the training of most mental health professionals. Many then continue to refine and perfect these skills over decades of clinical practice.

The generic psychosocial assessment has been outlined and written about in countless standard texts. In 2004 National Institute for Clinical Excellence (NICE) guidelines on self-harm were published by the UK Department of Health.[1] These indicate some general aims for assessing young people that have presented to services following self-harm.

In this chapter the emphasis is placed on highlighting and expanding the areas of the assessment that are of particular importance in cases of self-harm.

The TA outlined here is to be considered an augmentation of the psychosocial assessment as described by NICE. It is clear that the comprehensive and thorough history and examination of the patient has to form the basis of any subsequent, more therapeutically orientated psychological intervention.

The management of risk remains the key issue at the forefront of the clinicians mind. The aim being to optimise this by eliciting a collaborative approach with the patient, based on enhanced insight and curiosity on behalf of both the young person and assessor.

Some authors describe the ideal assessment as incorporating the use of specific risk assessment tools to supplement the usual assessment process and also better to inform clinical decision-making.[2] The usefulness of these tools has been questioned[3] and they certainly should not substitute for a comprehensive risk assessment. Relevant examples of these measures include:

1. The Suicide Intent Scale (SIS), developed by Beck *et al.* in 1974[4]
2. The Suicide Ideation Questionnaire (SIQ), developed by Reynolds in 1987[5]
3. The Brief Reasons for Living Inventory for Adolescents (BRFL-A), developed in 1996.[6]

These tools generally are not geared towards engaging the patient, increasing their insight or serving a therapeutic purpose. For these reasons, as well as the realistic constraints of what can be imposed on a young person under the circumstances, TA does not incorporate any such specific measures. Measures of suicidality and risk are discussed in more detail in Chapter 2 of this book.

Planning for the assessment

Some general principles that need to be considered before the assessment even begins are listed below.

a. *Where to conduct the assessment.* On most wards it will be possible to meet with the young person in a closed room that provides adequate privacy. In emergency departments (EDs) this can be a problem as space is often more limited and cubicles are usually screened only with a curtain. In addition to issues around privacy it is also important that the interview is not disturbed. Finally, for the purposes of the TA it is necessary to have a table on which the clinician can draw and write the formulation diagrams.

b. *Safety.* The safety of the clinician and also the patient must be considered carefully prior to starting the assessment. The patient is often unknown to staff and likely to be in a state of crisis, which can present a risk of unexpected and aggressive

(side margin) Assessment Manual

behaviour. Efforts should be made to gauge the level of anger, agitation, distress and unpredictability prior to inviting the patient into the interview room. This information can help to decide if a third person should join the clinician for the interview or simply be close by. It is always advisable to inform other members of staff where and when the interview is being conducted and also to determine if the room is equipped with a panic or emergency call button. Standard advice, such as sitting between the patient and the door, also applies to self-harm assessments.

c. *Who to see*. The issue of who to invite into the assessment can be a complicated one. Ideally part of the assessment would be alone with the patient and the other part would also include the parents or carers. Working with the family is explored in more detail in the chapter on systemic/family interventions. Often the parents/carers or the young person request to see the assessing clinician alone. If the patient makes this request then there are several issues that need to be considered, including the patient's age, mental capacity, the adult's legal status and the exact reasons given by the young person for their decision. For example, if they fear for their own safety at the hands of the adult.

d. *Capacity*. It may be necessary to clearly establish and document whether the young person has capacity to consent to the proposed treatments or investigations. This is of particular importance when there is a disagreement between the young person, their legal guardians and professionals about further management. In order to demonstrate capacity to consent to treatments or investigations the young person must be able to:

- understand the nature, purpose and possible consequences of investigations or treatments
- understand consequences of not having the investigations or treatments
- retain this information
- weigh this information in balance
- communicate the decision to others.

Note

At 16 years of age a young person can be presumed to have the capacity to consent and a young person under 16 years of age may have the capacity to consent, depending on their maturity and ability to understand the nature of the investigations or treatments.

In many UK hospitals it is standard procedure to inform social services in all hospital presentations of self-harm in under-18-year-olds. In view of this, it is often helpful to consult with the relevant social worker prior to the assessment in order to consider the possibility of conducting a joint assessment. If this is indicated, it can be more efficient and also helpful for both professionals involved. In such circumstances it is important to explain to patients that the involvement of social services is routine practice.

e. *Confidentiality.* Patients should be told that assessments are confidential unless it becomes apparent that there are clear risks to the patient's safety or the safety of others. Under these circumstances it may be necessary to breach their confidentiality. If this occurs then they will be informed and the reasons explained to them. Patients should also be informed that information is routinely shared between medical specialities, social services and also GPs, who adhere to the same code of confidentiality.

A particularly difficult situation may arise in a case of a young person refusing to share information about themselves with others, for example with the young person's parents. The information should be shared without consent in the following cases:

- when there is an overriding public interest in sharing the information
- when the disclosure is in the best interests of a child or young person who does not have capacity to make a decision about disclosure
- when disclosure is required by law.

In the case of a capacitous young person refusing to share information, such information could still be disclosed to the relevant persons or authorities if this is necessary to protect the child or young person, or someone else, from risk of death or serious harm.

Many areas involving capacity and confidentiality remain unclear and change over time. When dealing with these issues it is important to:

- seek senior advice
- seek legal advice
- clearly document all decisions and reasons for these decisions.

Before starting

It is necessary to obtain consent from the young person's parent or guardian and/or the young person themselves, before starting the psychosocial assessment. The outcome of this should then be documented in the medical records.

Engagement and rapport

After completing the necessary introductions, the following minutes with the patient can be particularly important in determining what will be accomplished during the assessment as a whole. This is because it is of great importance to establish a good rapport with the young person in order to gain their trust, enable them to relax and not feel that they are being judged or interrogated. This all helps to facilitate both information gathering and also the therapeutic components of the assessment.

An important early objective is to move the patient's presentation of self-harm from being a shameful experience to one that is dedicated to looking at 'how' and 'why' it occurred and what can be done to understand it. Patients may respond better if the therapist tries to understand their difficulties in the form of a story or narrative. Therapists will attempt to show how their problems represent the continuation of, or attempts to solve, past difficulties and must clarify what patients were and were not responsible for.

It may often be best to start talking about an area that is not directly related to the self-harming, such as the young person's interests and strengths and then find a way of linking this to challenges or problems.

It may be helpful to discover what thoughts, feelings and bodily sensations the patient had when they performed the self-harm, what it means for them and the motivation behind it, for example: pain, sight of blood, release of tension.

Content of assessment

The headings which follow are those commonly used to divide up a psychiatric history. It is assumed that the reader will have some knowledge of what is routinely covered by each of the headings, so that the comments which follow here are focused on important issues to expand in cases of self-harm.

Before meeting the patient basic demographic details should be clarified. These include the patient's sex, age, ethnicity, social situation and legal status. This information can be important in determining certain risk issues. It is known that self-harm is more common in adolescent girls.[7,8] Studies in the USA have shown that in a school sample of ethnically diverse adolescents, Pakistani children had a threefold elevated risk for a recent suicide attempt.[9] Another study showed an increased risk of attempted suicide in homeless young people.[10]

1. Circumstances of admission or history of presenting complaint

This must include a detailed description of the current self-harm, with a chronological account of the events surrounding any index self-harm incident. Areas to explore are discussed below.

Method

In general more violent methods of self-harm or attempted suicide are particularly worrying. Research has indicated that the likelihood of further suicide attempts and subsequent completed suicide is much greater after attempts of high medical

Assessment Manual

Assessment Manual

lethality, e.g. hanging, shooting or jumping,[11] and when there is escalating severity of self-harm.[12]

The most common methods of self-harming in the UK are drug overdoses and cutting.[7] The method is also important to explore in terms of how it relates to intent. For example if a firearm was used then there is likely to be less potential for ambivalence regarding the outcome on behalf of the patient.

On the other hand, an objectively less serious method must not be assumed to reflect less intent or a lower degree of desperation on the part of the patient. It may just be a reflection of the limited methods to which any young person has access.

Intent

This can sometimes be quite different from what is objectively seen as the lethality. For example, if someone takes a potentially fatal overdose but genuinely think it's just going to ensure that they sleep really well for the night. For this reason it is important to clarify what the person wanted to happen and what they believed would happen.

Some authors failed to find significant correlation between the lethality of the attempt and intent to die,[13] although generally the assessment of intent is regarded as a key component of risk assessment.[14,15]

Lethality

This is closely linked to the method and intent. The objective risk and danger the young person has exposed themselves to needs to be determined as well as subjective lethality. Any particular method may have a variable lethality depending on how it is carried out.

Objective medical lethality may not be a good discriminator of adolescent suicide attempters.[16] One study[17] pointed out that impulsive behaviour could result in an attempt of relatively high lethality with relatively low intent.

Other authors argue that in general medical seriousness of self-harm (objective lethality) may be determined by the interaction between suicidal intent and the young person's belief about the lethality of the act, i.e. subjective lethality.[2]

Precipitants

The assessor should clarify exactly what happened leading up to the self-harm. Typically there may have been a recent interpersonal conflict, loss, bereavement or similar incident. Stressful events that have been specifically linked to suicidal behaviour include falling out with parents and boyfriends/girlfriends, disciplinary crises like a recent or anticipated arrest or court appearance, or academic failure and punishment.[18,19] It has also been found that up to one-third are unable to identify a clear precipitant.[7,20]

Preparation/planning

Was the self-harm spontaneous or premeditated? In cases of the latter individuals may have stored up tablets in advance, or purchased razor blades. In more serious instances or unequivocal suicide attempts, there may have been a suicide note written, or intricate plans to avoid discovery.

High levels of impulsivity were found both in first-time attempters and repeat attempters.[21,22] This has been related to possible developing personality disorder. Some studies have shown that only 10–15 per cent of teenagers presenting to the ED reported thinking about their attempt for more than a day.[23–25]

Communication/precautions

Did the young person inform anyone of their self-harming actions, either before or afterwards? Were they likely to be found or seen?

Concurrent use of drugs or alcohol (see also Point 9 below)

Suicidal behaviour has a strong association with substance and alcohol misuse and so this part of the history should be explored in detail. Suicidal behaviour is often pre-dated by substance and alcohol misuse, and has been found in up to two-thirds of older boys.[26,27] In young people substance misuse is one of the predictors of subsequent suicidal behaviour.[28]

Remorse/reflection

It is very important to ask what the feelings and thoughts of the young person are in hindsight with respect to their self-harming behaviour. They may still feel like self-harming or even killing themselves and 'wish it would have worked'. The expression of hopelessness in the context of depressive symptomatology is a feature of both repeat attempts and worse prognosis.[29–31]

2. Past psychiatric history

Self-harm is a risk factor for further self-harm and also suicide. Twelve to 30 per cent of adolescent suicide attempters report having made a previous attempt.[32,33,7] About 40 per cent of completed suicides have made a previous known suicide attempt.[26,27]

Also, self-harm often occurs in the context of an altered mental state due to underlying mental illness. Almost all children and teenagers who commit suicide are suffering from a psychiatric disorder at the time they died.[26,27,34,35] Up to three quarters of adolescents who attempt suicide will have a mood disorder.[36,37,38] This is often comorbid with a conduct, anxiety or substance abuse disorder. Some studies have linked panic attacks with an increased risk of suicidal behaviour in adolescents.[39,40]

3. Medical history

Physical illness can act as a risk factor for suicidal behaviour in young people.[18] Therefore, it is important to enquire about any serious physical illness, either acute or chronic.

4. Drug history/allergies

Is the patient taking any prescription medication? Certain medicines can cause depression as a side effect and the SSRI (selective serotonin reuptake inhibitors) group of antidepressants themselves have been linked to causing suicidality, particularly in young people.[41] Access to tablets is a risk factor for taking overdoses so it is often advisable to take away a patient's medication.

5. Family history

The assessor should clarify exactly how the young person's immediate family is constituted. For example, who lives at home, who works and at what times, what are the relationships like at home. High levels of marital conflict and conflict between children and parents have been linked to young people who attempt suicide.[42–44] Suicide attempters are also more likely than control subjects to live in single-parent families.[45,46]

It is very important to establish if there is a family history of suicidal behaviour as this is a risk factor for completed suicide.[39,47–51]

The presence of parental psychopathology, depression and substance abuse in particular have been found to be associated with completed suicide[39,11,48] and also with adolescent suicidal ideation and attempts.[52–54]

6. Personal history/developmental history

Early childhood recollections of any history of trauma or abuse (emotional, physical or sexual), are likely to be highly relevant. Two longitudinal community studies have found self-reported child sexual abuse to be significantly associated with an increased risk of adolescent suicidal behaviour.[55,56] Similar evidence exists for physical abuse in childhood.

It can be useful to identify a disrupted background in terms of how often a young person has moved home, any past history of intra-familial conflicts, exposure to domestic violence, etc.

7. Psychosexual history

In homosexual young people there have been high rates of suicidal behaviour reported. Studies have found a two- to sixfold increase in risk of non-lethal suicidal behaviour for homosexual and bisexual youths.

Assessment Manual

8. Social history

The degree of psychosocial support, including friendships and relationships should be explored. In young people, as well as looking at the family's circumstances and functioning, there should be a closer examination of the situation at school, what achievements or problems have been experienced. Interestingly it has been demonstrated that bullying, both for the victim and the perpetrator, increases the risk for suicidal ideation.[57] Poor school or college attendance has also been linked to completed and attempted suicide.

There is established evidence for contagion/imitation being a significant factor in adolescent suicide. This relates to both suicide clusters and also the wider influence of mass media.

Compared with community controls youth suicide attempters have consistently been found to have higher rates of sociodemographic disadvantage.[58–60]

Individuals' coping styles and problem solving abilities have been studied with interesting outcomes. Poor interpersonal problem-solving ability has been reported to differentiate suicidal from non-suicidal youths.[23,61]

Other factors to explore include interests and hobbies, and methods of meeting needs.

9. Non-prescribed drug and alcohol use

In addition to asking about substance use at the time of the self-harm it is important to explore any previous history. One study showed that 16.7 per cent of adolescent suicides had an onset of substance abuse within 12 months of death.[63]

10. Forensic history

Previous violent or aggressive behaviour should be identified as well as any previous offences or convictions, especially if they occurred in the more recent past. The person could be facing an imminent court case. Research has shown that young suicide attempters are more hostile than control subjects.[63]

11. Mental state examination

It is of primary importance to identify any currently active psychiatric disorder such as depression or psychosis.

Many of the risk factors indicated and referenced above could be discovered and explored within the mental state examination.

The standard headings are given below.

Appearance and behaviour

This could include visible evidence of past and current self-harming behaviour like cuts and scars. It would be important to note the level of agitation and distress at the time of the assessment and also the degree of cooperation shown by the young person.

Speech

It is likely to be more difficult to both assess and engage a patient who is very withdrawn and uncommunicative. An incomplete assessment then makes it harder to determine risks.

Mood

If it has not been established earlier, then it is usually during the assessment of mood that a clinician might ask specific questions regarding current suicidality or self-harm ideation. This should involve exploring feelings, ideation, plans and intent. Depressed states of mind and particularly hopelessness in the context of depression were found to make adolescents more likely to attempt suicide.[64]

Biological symptoms of depression often indicate the presence of a depressive disorder and should not be forgotten.

Thoughts

Certain cognitive coping patterns have been linked to suicidal adolescents. In general, these can be seen as ineffective strategies or a failure to use appropriate coping strategies. The research in this area has used various definitions of coping and as a result it is harder to make general conclusions about this issue.

Predominantly negative and pessimistic thinking is of concern, especially in relation to the future. In some instances, such as psychotic depression or with active substance misuse, this type of thinking can take on a delusional intensity. If this or any other psychotic thought disturbance is evident then the level of risk is increased.

Perception

Quasi-psychotic experiences are common in the young people presenting with self-harm. These need to be differentiated from true hallucinations. Any psychotic symptoms that feature command auditory hallucinations to repeat self-harm or commit suicide are a serious concern, even if found in isolation with no further evidence of psychosis.

Cognition

In addition to establishing the young person's orientation and concentration, it can be helpful to clarify if the young person has clear memories of their self-harming behaviour or if it appears that they may have been acting in a more dissociated state.

Insight

It is useful to establish whether patients consider themselves to have a problem or to need help as this may be the first step towards successful engagement with services. Dropping out of treatment has been linked with poorer outcomes.[66]

It is crucial to remember that risk factors identified in the history can act in an accumulative manner. In view of this, it is necessary to explore as many areas as possible, even if certain significant risks become apparent early in an assessment.

Protective factors and reasons for living

Some of the information obtained in the history could be usefully identified as including important protective factors. Family cohesion has been reported as a protective factor for suicidal behaviour among adolescents.[67]

Other factors might include:

1. confiding and caring relationships
2. outside interests, including religious activities
3. good self-esteem
4 internal locus of control
5. positive school experience.

Risk assessment

A statement should be made regarding risk of harm to self and others based on the assessment and a weighing-up of the various risk factors and protective factors outlined above. This statement is often divided into mild, moderate and severe risk.

It can also be helpful to add the temporal (immediate, short-term or long-term) or situational perspective. For example, if a young person is currently being abused within the family and this is the acute cause of their self-harming behaviour then in the immediate term they could be at severe risk if they returned to this situation, but outside of this situation the risk could be low.

Clinical opinion/diagnosis

This would follow the usual format as in any other psychiatric assessment. In all cases of self-harm the clinical opinion should include a view on whether the patient needs to remain in hospital, either on a paediatric ward or a psychiatric inpatient unit. It is not always possible to arrive at a formal ICD-10 or DSM IV diagnosis but a preliminary formulation is helpful.

References

1. National Collaborating Centre for Mental Health. *Self-harm: the short-term physical and psychological management and secondary prevention of self-harm in primary*

Assessment Manual

and secondary care. Clinical Guideline 16. London: Gaskell & British Psychological Society; 2004.

2. Brown GK, Henriques GR, Sosdjan D, *et al*. Suicide intent and accurate expectations of lethality: predictors of medical lethality of suicide attempts. *J Consult Clin Psychol* 2004;72:1170–4.

3. Hjelmeland H, Hawton K, Nordvik H, *et al*. Why people engage in parasuicide: a cross-cultural study of intentions. *Suicide Life Threat Behav* 2002;32:380–93.

4. Beck AT, Schuyler D, Herman I. Development of suicidal intent scales. In: Beck AT, Resnick H, Lettieri D, editors. *The prediction of suicide*. Bowie MD: Charles Press; 1974: pp. 45–56.

5. Reynolds W. *Suicide Ideation Questionnaire*. Odessa, FL: Psychological Assessment Resources;1987.

6. Osman A, Kopper B, Barrios F, *et al*. The brief reasons for living inventory for adolescents – BRFL-A. *J Abnorm Child Psychol* 1996;24:433–43.

7. Hawton K, O'Grady J, Osborn M, *et al*. Adolescents who take overdoses: their characteristics, problems and contacts with helping agencies. *Br J Psychiatry* 1982;140:118–23.

8. Hawton K, Rodham K, Evans E, *et al*. Deliberate self-harm in adolescents: self report survey in schools in England. *BMJ* 2002;325:1207–11.

9. Roberts RE, Chen YR, Roberts CR. Ethnocultural differences in prevalence of adolescent suicidal behaviours. *Suicide Life Threat Behav* 1997;27:208–17.

10. Votta E, Manion I. Suicide, high-risk behaviors, and coping style in homeless adolescent males' adjustment. *J Adolesc Health* 2004;34:237–43.

11. Brent DA, Perper JA, Goldstein CE, *et al*. Risk factors for adolescent suicide: a comparison of adolescent suicide victims with suicidal inpatients. *Arch Gen Psychiatry* 1988;45:581–8.

12. Carter G, Reith DM, Whyte IM, *et al*. Repeated self-poisoning: increasing severity of self-harm as a predictor of subsequent suicide. *Br J Psychiatry* 2005;186:253–7.

13. Plutchik R, van Praag H, Picard S, *et al*. Is there a relation between the seriousness of suicidal intent and the lethality of the suicide attempt? *Psychiatry Res* 1989;27:71–9.

14. Harriss L, Hawton K, Zahl D. Value of measuring suicidal intent in the assessment of people attending hospital following self-poisoning or self-injury. *Br J Psychiatry* 2005;186(1):60–6

15. Brown GK, Henriques GR, Sosdjan D, Beck AT. Suicide intent and accurate expectations of lethality: predictors of medical lethality of suicide attempts. *J Consult Clin Psychol* 2004;72(6):1170–4.

16. Spirito A, Overholser J, Stark L. Common problems and coping strategies, II: Findings with adolescent suicide attempters. *J Abnorm Child Psychol* 1989;17:213–21.

17. Brent D. Practitioner Review: The aftercare of adolescents with deliberate self-harm. *J Child Psychol Psychiatry* 1997;38:277–86.

18. Lewinsohn PM, Rhode P, Seeley JR. Adolescent suicidal ideation and attempts: prevalence, risk factors, and clinical implications. *Clin Psychol* 1996;3:25–46.

19. Beautrais AL, Joyce PR, Mulder RT. Precipitating factors and life events in serious suicide attempts among youths aged thirteen through twenty-four years. *J Am Acad Child Adolesc Psychiatry* 1997;36:1543–51.

20. Kienhorst CW, de Wilde EJ, Diekstra RF, *et al*. Adolescents' image of their suicide attempt. *J Am Acad Child Adolesc Psychiatry* 1995;34:623–8.

Assessment Manual

21. Stein D, Apter A, Ratzoni G, *et al*. Association between multiple suicide attempts and negative affects in adolescents. *J Am Acad Child Adolesc Psychiatry* 1998;37:488–94.

22. Kingsbury S, Hawton K, Steinhardt K, *et al*. Do adolescents who take overdoses have specific psychological characteristics: a comparative study with psychiatric and community controls. *J Am Acad Child Adolesc Psychiatry* 1999;38:1125–31.

23. Rotheram-Borus MJ, Trautman PD, Dopkins SC, *et al*. Cognitive style and pleasant activities among female adolescent suicide attempters. *J Consult Clin Psychol* 1990;58:554–61.

24. Piacentini J, Rotheram-Borus MJ, Trautman P, *et al*. Psychosocial correlates of treatment compliance in adolescent suicide attempters. Presented at the Association for Advancement of Behaviour Therapy Meeting 1991, New York, ABCT;1991.

25. Negron R, Piacentini J, Graae F, *et al*. Microanalysis of adolescent suicide attempters and ideators during the acute suicidal episode. *J Am Acad Child Adolesc Psychiatry* 1997;36:1512–19.

26. Shaffer P, Gould MS, Fisher P, Trautman *et al*. Psychiatric diagnosis in child and adolescent suicide. *Arch Gen Psychiatry* 1996;53:339–48.

27. Brent DA, Baugher M, Bridge J, *et al*. Age- and sex-related risk factors for adolescent suicide. *J Am Acad Child Adolesc Psychiatry* 1999;38:1497–505.

28. Borowsky IW, Ireland M, Resnick MD. Adolescent suicide attempts: risks and protectors. *Pediatrics* 2001;107:485–93.

29. Kienhorst CW, de Wilde EJ, Diekstra RF, *et al*. Differences between adolescent suicide attempters and depressed adolescents. *Acta Psychiatr Scand* 1992;85:222–8.

30. Morano CD, Cisler RA, Lemerond J. Risk factors for adolescent suicidal behaviour: loss, insufficient familial support, and hopelessness. *Adolescence* 1993;28:851–65.

31. Steer RA, Kumar G, Beck AT. Self-reported suicidal ideation in adolescent psychiatric inpatients. *J Consult Clin Psychol* 1993;61:1096–9.

32. White HC. Self-poisoning in adolescents. *Br J Psychiatry* 1974;124:24–35.

33. Rohn RD, Sarles RM, Kenney TJ, *et al*. Adolescents who attempt suicide. *J Pediatr* 1977;90:636–8.

34. Marttunen MJ, Aro HM, Henriksson MM *et al*. Mental disorders in adolescent suicide: DSM-III-R axes I and II diagnoses in suicides among thirteen- to nineteen-year olds in Finland. *Arch Gen Psychiatry* 1991;48:834–9.

35. Marttunen MJ, Henriksson MM, Aro HM, *et al*. Suicide among female adolescents: characteristics and comparison with males in the age group thirteen to twenty-two years. *J Am Acad Child Adolesc Psychiatry* 1995;34:1297–307.

36. Andrews JA, Lewinsohn PM. Suicidal attempts among older adolescents: prevalence and co-occurrence with psychiatric disorders. *J Am Acad Child Adolesc Psychiatry* 1992;31:655–62.

37. Beautrais AL, Joyce PR, Mulder RT. Psychiatric illness in a New Zealand sample of young people making serious suicide attempts. *N Z Med J* 1998;111:44–8.

38. Gould MS, King R, Greenwald S, *et al*. Psychopathology associated with suicidal ideation and attempts among children and adolescents. *J Am Acad Child Adolesc Psychiatry* 1998;37:915–23.

39. Gould MS, Fisher P, Parides M, *et al*. Psychosocial risk factors of child and adolescent completed suicide. *Arch Gen Psychiatry* 1996;53:1155–62.

40. Pilowsky DJ, Wu L, Anthony JC. Panic attacks and suicide attempts in mid-adolescence. *Am J Psychiatry* 1999;156:1545–9.

41. Hammad T, Laughren T, Racoosin J. Suicidality in pediatric patients treated with antidepressant drugs. *Arch Gen Psychiatry* 2006;63:332–9.

42. Taylor EA, Stansfield SA. Children who poison themselves. I. A clinical comparison with psychiatric controls. *Br J Psychiatry* 1984;145:127–32.

43. Trautman PD, Shaffer D. Treatment of child and adolescent suicide attempters. In: Sudak HS, Ford AB, Rushforth NB, editors. *Suicide in the young.* Boston: John Wright-PSG; 1984.

44. Asarnow JR. Suicidal ideation and attempts during middle childhood: associations with perceived family stress and depression among child psychiatric inpatients. *J Clin Child Psychol* 1992;55:361–6.

45. Groholt B, Ekeberg O, Wichstrom L, *et al.* Young suicide attempters: a comparison between a clinical and an epidemiological sample. *J Am Acad Child Adolesc Psychiatry* 2000;39:868–75.

46. Wichstrom L. Predictors of adolescent suicide attempters: a nationally representative longitudinal study of Norwegian adolescents. *J Am Acad Child Adolesc Psychiatry* 2000;39:603–10.

47. Agerbo E, Nordentoft M, Mortensen PB. Familial, psychiatric, and socioeconomic risk factors for suicide in young people: nested case control study. *BMJ* 2002;325:74.

48. Brent DA, Perper JA, Moritz G, *et al.* Familial risk factors for adolescent suicide: a case-control study. *Acta Psychiatr Scand* 1994;89:52–8.

49. Brent DA, Bridge J, Johnson BA, *et al.* Suicidal behavior runs in families: a controlled family study of adolescent suicide victims. *Arch Gen Psychiatry* 1996;53:1145–52.

50. Shaffer D. Suicide in childhood and early adolescence. *J Child Psychol Psychiatry* 1974;15:275–91.

51. Shafii M, Carrigan S, Wittinghill J, *et al.* Psychological autopsy of completed suicide in children and adolescents. *Am J Psychiatry* 1985;142:1061–4.

52. Fergusson DM, Lynskey M. Childhood circumstances, adolescent adjustment, and suicide attempts in a New Zealand birth cohort. *J Am Acad Child Adolesc Psychiatry* 1995;34:612–22.

53. Joffe RT, Offord DR, Boyle MH. Ontario Child Health Study: suicidal behavior in youth aged 12–16 years. *Am J Psychiatry* 1988;145:1420–3.

54. Kashani JH, Goddard P, Reid JC. Correlates of suicidal ideation in a community sample of children and adolescents. *J Am Acad Child Adolesc Psychiatry* 1989;28:912–17.

55. Fergusson DM, Horwood LJ, Lynskey MT. Childhood sexual abuse and psychiatric disorder in young adulthood, II: psychiatric outcomes of childhood sexual abuse. *J Am Acad Child Adolesc Psychiatry* 1996;35:1365–74.

56. Silverman AB, Reinherz HZ, Giaconia RN. The long-term sequelae of child and adolescent abuse: a longitudinal community study. *Child Abuse Negl* 1996;20:709–23.

57. Kaltiala-Heino R, Rimpela M, Marttunen M, *et al.* Bullying, depression, and suicidal ideation in Finnish adolescents: school survey. *BMJ* 1999;319:348–51.

58. Beautrais AL, Joyce PR, Mulder RT. Risk factors for serious suicide attempts among youths aged 13 through 24 years. *J Am Acad Child Adolesc Psychiatry* 1996;35:1174–82.

59. Fergusson DM, Woodward LJ, Horwood LJ. Risk factors and life processes associated with the onset of suicidal behaviour during adolescence and early adulthood. *Psychol Med* 2000;30:23–39.

60. Wunderlich U, Bronisch T, Wittchen HU. Comorbidity patterns in adolescents and young adults with suicide attempts. *Eur Arch Psychiatry Clin Neurosci* 1998;248:87–95.

61. Asarnow JR, Carlson GA, Guthrie D. Coping strategies, self-perceptions, hopelessness, and perceived family environments in depressed suicidal children. *J Consult Clin Psychol* 1987;55:361–6.
62. Brent D, Perper J, Moritz G, *et al.* Psychiatric risk factors for adolescent suicide: A case-control study. *J Am Acad Child Adolesc Psychiatry* 1993;32:521–9.
63. Simonds J, McMahon T, Armstrong D. Youth suicide attempters compared with a control group: psychological, affective and attitudinal variables. *Suicide Life Threat Behav* 1991;21:134–51.
64. Dori G, Overholser J. Depression, hopelessness and self-esteem: accounting for suicidality in adolescent psychiatric patients. *Suicide Life Threat Behav* 1999;29:309–18.
65. Litt IF, Cuskey WR, Rudd S. Emergency room evaluation of the adolescent who attempts suicide: compliance with follow-up. *J Adolesc Health Care* 1983;4:106–8.
66. McKeown RE, Garrison CZ, Cuffe SP, *et al.* Incidence and predictors of suicidal behaviors in a longitudinal sample of young adolescents. *J Am Acad Child Adolesc Psychiatry* 1998;37:612–19.

Assessment Manual

CHAPTER 12

DEVELOPING UNDERSTANDING

Dennis Ougrin

Introduction

One way to start therapeutic assessment (TA) is to ask the young person:

Key question

How would you know that this assessment had been useful after we've finished?

A very common answer to this question is: 'I would like to understand what has happened', or 'I would like to be less confused about it all'.

Although this sounds like a tall order, developing a joint understanding of the young person's difficulties is one of the key tasks of TA. In order to develop this understanding TA uses diagrams derived from cognitive analytic therapy. Each diagram consists of three main elements:

- reciprocal roles
- core pain
- procedures.

It would probably be unwise to offer these terms to the young person during TA. For the purposes of this manual, we will briefly explain each element and how they can be linked in a diagram.

Reciprocal roles

What are reciprocal roles?

> *Reciprocal roles are difficult to understand, but once understood they become a very useful tool not just in TA but also in other aspects of therapeutic work. Reciprocal roles are seen as central to the diagram. They provide a way of trying to understand the origin of the young person's difficulties.*

Reciprocal roles could be described as:

- patterns of relationships
- ways of being with others
- power alignments with others.

Reciprocal roles are *derived from the early experiences* of the young person, principally with parents but also with other important figures: a young person who was frequently criticised by a parent and only rarely praised for achieving may learn to criticise others, perhaps to avoid being criticised.

Reciprocal roles are *internalised*: a young person who was frequently criticised by a parent is likely to frequently criticise herself.

Reciprocal roles are frequently *polarised*: a young person might frequently occupy two extreme positions: either being criticised or criticising others. It is like being stuck in the lift with only the top and the bottom buttons working.

Reciprocal roles may have been useful in the past but may have become *dysfunctional* in later adolescence: switching from criticising to being criticised may have been adaptive in an early environment but may cause problems for example in forming relationships or friendships.

Reciprocal roles are *persistent*. Despite causing problems reciprocal roles may remain unrevised for a long time – switching from criticising to being criticised may be unpleasant but it will be familiar.

The reciprocal roles available to a young person presenting with self-harm may be *limited* in their repertoire.

Reciprocal roles are particularly liable to being *activated at times of distress* – all of us might have experienced acting like our parents would have done especially in stressful situations.

Key question

Tell me what was going on before you thought of harming yourself?

> *When did things start to go wrong?*
> *What was it that upset you most?*
> *What was it that pressed your buttons?*
> *What did you do?/How did you respond?*
> *What did other people do?/How did they respond?*
> *How did it feel?*
> *What do you think other people felt?*
> *Have you experienced (the possible reciprocal role, e.g. being rejected) before?*
> *When/where/who else was involved?*

> *Have you experienced (the possible reciprocal role, e.g. being criticised) during this assessment today?*
> *It seems you may have felt like being (the possible reciprocal role e.g. being misunderstood) today*
> *It seems you may have been (the possible reciprocal role e.g. criticizing others) in response to how others made you feel*

The four principal sources of reciprocal roles are:

1. interactions with professionals
2. interactions with carers
3. similar episodes in the past (history)
4. events leading to self-harm.

You could try to get the young person to describe the relationship patterns, i.e. how things usually are. In practice it is easier to get a description of a specific episode, like an instance of self-harming.

Interactions with professionals

Let's consider the following example. During TA a young person may tell you that there is no point in this assessment and that all psychiatrists are rubbish. This might be interpreted as the young person trying to occupy the **critical/rejecting** pole in the **rejecting–rejected** and **criticising–criticised** reciprocal role repertoire. You could then respond in several ways.

1. Start justifying yourself and others (i.e. align yourself with a **criticised/rejected** position)
2. Respond angrily: 'If you feel this way, then of course this assessment is going to be a waste of time' (i.e. try to occupy the **rejecting/criticising** pole)
3. Use this material to further your understanding of the young person's difficulties: 'It sounds like you are frustrated and angry at the moment'.

The last response will be seen as the most productive way forward with a mental note to remember a possible reciprocal role procedure in operation.

Observing the young person occupying the **criticising/rejecting** position suggests he/she is trying to avoid being **rejected** or **criticised** – although, paradoxically, this in fact becomes a lot more likely. Young people frequently describe their experience in the emergency department (ED) as being one of rejection and humiliation at the hands of others.

Although the concept of reciprocal roles is complex, it is fairly easy to explain to a young person:

If you felt **rejected** and **abandoned** (or **controlled** or **invaded** etc.) many times in the past, you then become sensitive to these experiences. You may end up flipping into the opposite extremes of **rejecting, abandoning, controlling** or **invading**, etc., others to deal with the anxiety and hurt you feel. You may also end up hurting yourself as a way of dealing with these feelings.

Noting reciprocal roles during the one-to-one interview is one way of discovering them. Here we will describe three more ways of identifying reciprocal roles.

Interaction with the carer

Mother: *'I'm sick and tired of your behaviour, I can't cope with you any more'* (**abandoning**) Daughter (crying):*'I can't do anything to please you'* (**abandoned**)

Similar episodes in the past (history)

Look for evidence of repetitive patterns of relationships experienced by the young person throughout the history. Consider an example below.

Extract from history (Sabine)

Sabine remembers her mother to have always been unhappy with the quality of her school work (**criticising**), making her do homework over and over again until it was perfect (**controlling**). Sabine would then feel unmotivated and frustrated (**criticised, controlled**)

The main themes emerging from this history are the reciprocal roles of:

- **criticising** in relation to being **criticised** and
- **controlling** in relation to being **controlled**.

They are depicted in the way shown in Figure 12.1.

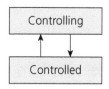
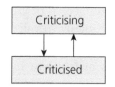

Figure 12.1 Reciprocal roles.

It is important to consider two issues here:

- You can only propose this pattern as a theory and without attributing blame to anyone. The development of reciprocal roles is always an interpersonal process and children with certain developmental characteristics may be more likely to evoke particular responses from their guardians. For instance, hyperactive children may be more likely to evoke criticising and rejecting enactment of their parents' reciprocal roles. Conversely, children with greater emotional stability may develop adaptive ways of responding to the enactment of their parents' problematic reciprocal roles, even if this occurs frequently.

For example: *'It sounds like you have been feeling* **controlled/criticised** *a lot in the past'* is a neutral statement unlike *'It sounds like your mother has been* **criticising** *and* **controlling** *you all your life'*.

- The reciprocal role patterns always have interpsychic components (the young person may occupy either of the poles in relation to other people) and intrapsychic components (the young person may occupy either of the poles in relation to themselves). Self-harm is an example of **attacking/rejecting** the self, but could also be an example of **attacking/rejecting** others or an attempt to regain control over one's own self.

Events leading to self-harm

We will continue the example of Sabine here.

Sabine presented to the emergency department (ED) after an overdose. The overdose was precipitated by an argument between Sabine and her parents with the background of fears relating to poor exam results. Sabine felt under constant, albeit subtle, pressure to perform at her private school and was made to feel responsible for the family investment of a lot of money and effort into her education (parents **criticising** and **controlling**). The immediate reason for the argument with her parents was a disagreement over Sabine's going out to a gig. The parents at first agreed and then changed their minds saying Sabine was too tired and had to spend more time preparing for her exams (parents **controlling**). This provoked an angry reaction with Sabine crying, throwing things (Sabine **controlled**) and making vague threats of suicide that mother became very upset about (Sabine **controlling**). After the overdose mother was feeling very inadequate and guilty and thought she was a bad mother (mother **criticised** and **criticising** herself).

Let's look at another example.

Michelle presented with an overdose after her boyfriend dumped her (**rejected, abandoned**). The boyfriend also mocked Michelle for her distress after the break up. This added to Michelle's feeling of 'there is no point'. Michelle then took an overdose (**rejecting** and **abandoning** self).

History

Her biological parents had split up a few years earlier and there was an acrimonious divorce marred by violence. Michelle remembered being frequently left with relatives and sometimes she had been looked after by the local authorities during her childhood as her mother could not cope (**abandoned**). Her mother developed depression after the divorce and was repeatedly asking Michelle to stay with the

Assessment Manual

grandparents as Michelle's behaviour was making her depression worse (**abandoning, rejecting**). The relationship with her stepfather is difficult to the point of Michelle leaving home and staying with her best friend (**rejecting, abandoning**).

The main reciprocal roles elicited from this history are shown in Figure 12.2.

Figure 12.2 Reciprocal roles from Michelle's history.

The final brief history is that of Teresa. Teresa developed a brief and very intense homosexual relationship with the subject of a long-term infatuation she had (**ideally caring–ideally cared for**). After a break up, she stalked her ex-girlfriend (**attacking**). The ex-girlfriend alerted the police and had an injunction issued against Teresa. This led to Teresa withdrawing from social interactions and self-harming daily (**attacking** self–**attacked**).

The main reciprocal roles are shown in Figure 12.3.

Figure 12.3 Reciprocal roles from Teresa's history.

Examples of some other core reciprocal roles in young people presenting with self-harm are shown in Table 12.1.

Table 12.1 Core reciprocal roles

Parent derived	Child derived
Critical	Criticised
Controlling	Controlled
Abandoning	Abandoned
Rejecting	Rejected
Ideally caring	Ideally cared for
Betraying	Betrayed
Fusing	Fused with
Invading	Invaded
Judging	Judged

If the young person refuses to accept that she ever enacts any of the 'unacceptable' or 'angry' poles of reciprocal roles with other people (e.g. 'I am never rejecting or critical of others'), they may genuinely not be aware of these reciprocal roles and may discover them later. You could leave the reciprocal roles unfinished. In some cases young people may have learned to repress the 'unacceptable' poles in the reciprocal roles. The intrapsychic component would then usually be prominent – young people would generally accept that self-harm is an attack or rejection of the self. If you really want to push it, consider bringing the internalised abuser in. Careful though, as too much psychoanalysis can be bad for your blood pressure.

Younger children

If it seems likely that the young person may not be developmentally or situationally ready for these rather complex explorations it is sufficient to agree on a trigger – an event that commonly leads to activation of negative feelings or negative thoughts. The triggers frequently have an interpersonal nature reflecting the underlying reciprocal roles – bullying, being told off, being unfairly criticised, arguing or being called names are common examples.

Core pain

The core pain is the second essential part of the diagram. Core pain is a similar concept to the concept of core beliefs in cognitive therapy and includes the thoughts, feelings, ideas and images the young person has about themselves. The core pain is usually placed at the centre of the diagram and is seen as a result of enacting the reciprocal roles over time. For example, frequent experiences of **rejecting–rejected** reciprocal roles may lead to viewing the self as unlovable and unlikeable; **criticising–criticised** may lead to 'inadequate' or 'stupid' core pain, **ideally caring–ideally cared for** to 'hopeless' or 'lustful' core pain.

In the early work on TA these descriptions were avoided as they seemed to add to the negative emotions experienced by the young person during assessment. The 'as if' prefix may be added to indicate that these terms as not seen as absolute and there is potential for hope and change.

Key question

When you were/perceived being (describe reciprocal role or trigger) what thoughts did you have about yourself?

The best way to enquire about the core pain is to follow the young person's feelings and thoughts after the enactment of a reciprocal role.

> *What was going through your mind?*
> *What else went through your mind when you were most distressed?*

Assessment Manual

> *What did it mean to you?*
> *What images/memories did you have?*
> *What did you feel about yourself?*
> *Some people feel as if (possible core pain). Did you feel as if you were (possible core pain)?*

Example of Sabine (Figure 12.4)

Therapist: *When you are controlled or criticised, what thoughts do you have about yourself?*

Sabine: *As if I am stupid and inadequate.*

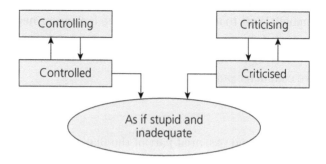

Figure 12.4 Sabine's example.

Example of Michelle (Figure 12.5)

Therapist: When you felt rejected and abandoned by your boyfriend, how did it make you feel about yourself?

Michelle: I felt as if there was no point, as if no one will ever love me or like me.

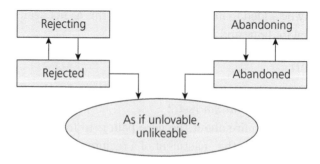

Figure 12.5 Michelle's example.

Example of Teresa (Figure 12.6)

Therapist: What thoughts about yourself did you have before taking the overdose?

Teresa: I felt lustful, dirty, as if I deserved punishment. I thought I would never be able to have a normal relationship.

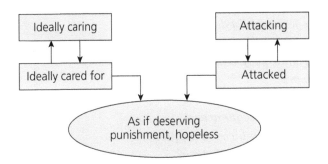

Figure 12.6 Teresa's example.

Younger children (Figure 12.7)

If a young person finds it difficult to describe any negative thoughts, try to identify feelings linked to specific triggers:

Therapist: When you are bullied how does it make you feel?

Young person: It makes me feel bad.

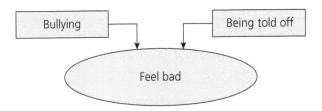

Figure 12.7 Younger children.

Procedures

> *Procedures are defined as maladaptive patterns of behaviour that inevitably lead to the reinforcement of the core pain, or feed into it. In TA the main procedures are drawn in a circular fashion, starting and ending with the core pain.*

The best way to draw a procedural sequence is to look in detail at the index episode of self-harm or other episodes where reciprocal roles and core pain ideas are activated.

Key question

When you are (describe core pain or reciprocal role) what happens next? What happens after that?

Try to get the young person to describe the usual patterns. If this is too difficult, tie this question in with a specific situation, like the time of self-harm.

> *What do you usually do next?*
> *What do you want to achieve?*
> *What do other people do?*
> *Does it work?*
> *What happens next?*
> *What are the consequences?*
> *What are the long-term consequences?*
> *How does it leave you feeling?*
> *How does it leave other people feeling?*
> *On the day of the overdose you felt controlled and unfairly criticised. What happened next?*
> *When you think of yourself as being worthless or unlovable what do you do next? What happens next?*

If the young person comes up with an exit at this point (e.g. when I feel horrible I go upstairs and listen to music) – note this valuable information. If the young person has difficulties describing the procedure offer some tentative ideas:

> *On the basis of what you described, it seems like one way you react to criticism and feeling not good enough is by trying to do everything perfectly.*
>
> *When you follow the procedure keep the following in mind: can you use the points identified as targets for the future work, i.e. can you imagine exits instead of the stages of the procedure. Ideally the more points of possible intervention you can identify the more useful the diagram.*
>
> *Figures 12.8–12.10 describe the procedural analysis.*

The following are some examples of common procedures that may be used to aid building the diagram.

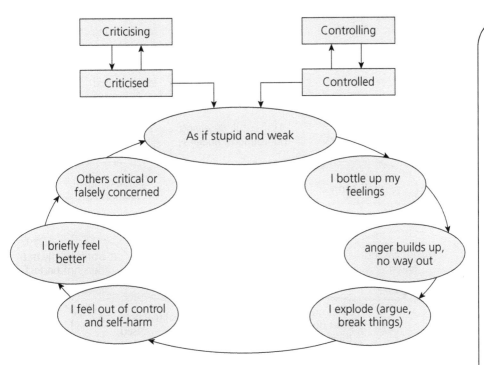

Figure 12.8 Sabine's diagram

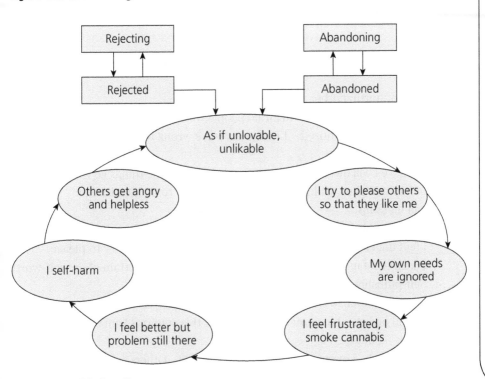

Figure 12.9 Michelle's diagram.

Assessment Manual

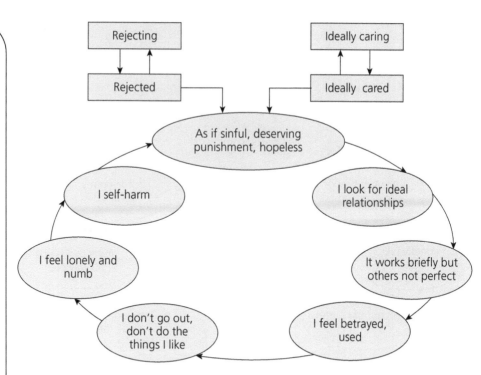

Figure 12.10 Teresa's diagram.

Examples of frequently encountered procedures

1. Fear of hurting other people's feelings:
   It's wrong to be angry – I'm afraid people will be hurt – I don't express feelings – I feel ignored/abused – I feel angry – It's wrong to be angry
2. Negative thinking:
   I believe I will mess up – I do things and some of the things go wrong – I dwell on my mistakes, which makes me more likely to make mistakes – I believe I will mess up
3. Trying to please:
   I feel uncertain of my self-worth – I want to be liked – I try to please – They take advantage – I feel angry and a failure - I feel uncertain of my self-worth
4. Self-punishment:
   I believe I am bad weak or guilty – I feel agitated, upset and out of control – I harm myself – I feel briefly relieved, but this confirms I am bad, weak, guilty
5. Upset feelings:
   I feel upset – I express my feelings explosively – Others feel attacked/rejected – Others attack/reject me – I feel upset

6. Perfectionist trap:

I feel 'not good enough' I try to be perfect – It's impossible and stressful – I make mistakes – I feel a failure – I feel I will never be perfect - I feel not good enough

7. Need of perfect care (1):

I feel I need attention/care/trust - I seek someone I can admire/perfectly care for/trust, who will admire/perfectly care for/trust me – It feels good until they fail – I feel they betrayed/rejected/abandoned – I hate that person - I feel I need attention/care/trust

8. Need of perfect care (2):

I feel I need attention/care/trust - I feel contemptuous/angry/suspicious – I reject them first to avoid being hurt – I feel lost, alone – I seek a new relationship - I feel I need attention/care/trust

9. Controlling others trap (1):

I feel I have no control – I seek someone to control – I manipulate/bully them to giving in – I feel good until they rebel or fail to comply – I feel angry and abandoned - I feel I have no control

10. Controlling others trap (2):

I feel I have no control – I manipulate/bully others to give in – they become obedient, crushed – I lose respect and lose interest – I feel lonely – I feel I have no control

11. Getting my needs met trap:

I have a need – I demand it in all or nothing way – others feel defensive – they agree initially but feel they can lose face – they change their mind – I feel angry – I have a need.

Younger children (Figure 12.11)

If a young person finds it difficult to describe long behavioural sequences, try to follow their descriptions:

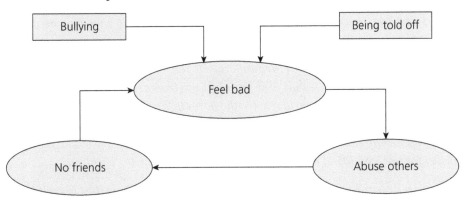

Figure 12.11 Diagram for younger children.

Assessment Manual

Therapist:	When you feel bad what do you do then?
Young person:	I tell them to piss off.
Therapist:	What happens next?
Young person:	Nothing. I have no friends left.

Practice exercise

Please have a look at this abridged history and draw a possible diagram. The authors' diagram is presented below; try to draw your own first and compare it with the one offered by the authors.

> *Rebecca is a 14-year-old White British young lady who lives with her parents and two younger sisters and is attending a strict religious school. Rebecca presented to the ED accompanied by her mother following an overdose. Rebecca felt miserable after an argument with her mother. She felt guilty and awkward after her mother said she couldn't speak to Rebecca in order not to upset her and risk self-harm. Rebecca wrote a 'goodbye' letter to her best friend then took approximately 16 paracetamol tablets that she found at home.*

Rebecca's view: the crucial point is the relationship between mother and Rebecca. Rebecca considers her mother to be constantly trying to control her, setting rules in a controlling manner, getting angry and arguing with her and rarely giving good enough explanations for the rules. She also feels that mother is accusing her of being defiant and not loving her parents.

Mother's view: Rebecca has difficulties in her relationships with most members of her family, although she is doing very well at school and has many friends. Rebecca would frequently defy the rules and would be contemptuous to her mother. Mother would usually lose the argument but would try to impose a punishment that Rebecca would disobey as well. This would lead mother to feel stupid, ineffective and contemptible and cause her to avoid spending any time with Rebecca – as if walking on eggshells.

There is a history of regular arguments in the family mainly between the parents, involving both verbal and physical confrontation. From a young age Rebecca would frequently try to resolve the parents' arguments that she perceived as stupid and would find herself on the receiving end of the parents' anger, both accusing her of interfering with their business. The parents would later feel guilty for not providing a good enough environment for the children.

There is a 2-year history of self-harm (cutting). Rebecca described herself being in an 'altered' state immediately prior to self-harm. She remembered that the most likely trigger of self-harm is arguing with her mother and feeling lonely and confused after the arguments when on her own in her bedroom. She thought the reasons for the arguments were around the perceived overcontrolling and overcritical actions of her mother (Figure 12.12).

In this diagram the following therapeutic targets could be highlighted:

1. relationship with mother
2. self-harming behaviour
3. negative ideas about self
4. isolating behaviour
5. enacting reciprocal roles.

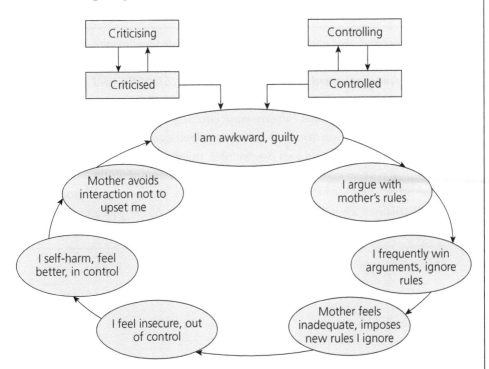

Figure 12.12 Author's version of the diagram.

Understanding Letter

The final tool derived from CAT is the 'Understanding Letter'. This is called the reformulation letter in CAT, but for the purposes of TA, the 'Understanding Letter' must contain not only the diagram but also the possible exits, targets and an encouragement towards further work. The 'Understanding Letters' will be presented at the end of some of the chapters describing specific exits.

Building the diagram algorithm

1. Identify and draw reciprocal roles (or triggers in younger adolescents) on the basis of
   - Events leading to self-harm
   - History
   - The young person's interaction with others
   - Your interaction with the young person
2. Identify and draw core pain (thoughts and/or associated feelings)
3. Identify a procedure starting and ending with core pain
4. Use the young person's descriptions as much as possible throughout
5. Check with the young person if the diagram makes sense.

In summary, this chapter describes how a joint understanding is developed in TA. The CAT-based diagram is constructed with identified reciprocal roles feeding into the core pain and giving rise to problematic procedures – patterns of behaviour that may have been useful once but are now causing distress and lead to self-harm. The diagrams are constructed using the young person's descriptions and may to a degree also involve different members of the family or even significant others. Diagrams provide a basis for identifying and trying to understand the young person's difficulties. They also provide a starting point for possible therapeutic change.

CHAPTER 13

INSTILLING HOPE

Dennis Ougrin

Introduction

Once you have identified a possible vicious cycle, it is important to start thinking about how to offer the young person a way forward.

Basically, all three main parts of the diagram could be targeted (identifying and changing reciprocal roles, core pain and procedures). The rest of this manual will describe how various ideas and techniques could be employed to break the cycles identified. This chapter highlights various techniques aimed at instilling hope, although of course the process of instilling hope begins from the very first question in the assessment.

Hopelessness is frequently associated with the young person feeling confused and overwhelmed. Developing an understanding of the young person's difficulties is the first step towards instilling hope. The next step is setting a target problem.

Target problem

Setting targets is a powerful way to instil hope. This could be seen as a move from chaos to structure and from hopelessness to hopefulness.

There isn't a right or wrong way of describing the target problem for the purposes of therapeutic assessment (TA). Different techniques described in this manual could result in identifying targets and so there is no need to force the young person or the family to do it at the beginning of the TA.

The target problem should ideally be linked to the diagram. Most young people like the analogy between the diagram and a chain: if we could break one link in the chain, the whole chain falls apart. Ask the young person to help you.

Key questions

You have helped me to understand your difficulties better by drawing this diagram. What do you think is the best target in the diagram?
What is the most important target?
What target may be the easiest to deal with?

Assessment Manual

Of course, if the young person feels confused and overwhelmed, it may not be possible to establish this focal point at all. In other cases a target problem could be formulated right at the end of the session. The following questions may help identify target problems (please also refer to Chapter 15 for the preferred future questions).

- If there was one thing you would like to change about yourself what would this one thing be?
- If I could grant you one wish (or three wishes if you feel particularly omnipotent), what would you like to change about yourself?
- How would you know that things have started to get better?

As always in this manual it is urged that therapists keep as close as possible to the young person's language. It is much better to have an imperfect target problem proposed by the young person than the most elegant one forced by the therapist.

Here are some examples of target problems; you will see that most of them are concretely related to the links in the procedural chains.

> *I want to stop being miserable*
> *I don't want to go crazy every time X happens*
> *I'd like to get along with X better*
> *How can I keep friends without ignoring my own needs (careful, do they want to become a psychotherapist?)*
> *I want to stop cutting (rare, if this is the target problem you ought to congratulate the young person for making this very important step. You could also congratulate yourself secretly, because the task of engaging this young person has just become a lot easier)*
> *I want to stop smoking dope (rare, again very specific and a workable target problem)*
> *F*** off, I don't know what you are talking about (fortunately also rare; prepare to get in touch with your Zen).*

You will see that the above examples are all 'I' statements reflecting the internal locus of control. Some young people might find it difficult to think in these terms and their targets could be different:

> *My mum has to stop nagging me*
> *My dad must spend more time with the family*
> *My boyfriend has to love me again.*

It is important to acknowledge these targets as legitimate and important for young people. However, if the object of change (mother, boyfriend, etc.) is not present at the assessment and there is no way of knowing what they think about this target, a subtle difference of emphasis needs to be introduced.

> *Even if your mother did not stop nagging you, how would you know that things were getting better?*
> *What could be done to make your dad more likely to spend time with the family?*
> *If you did get back together with your ex-boyfriend what difference would it make?*

Key question

Am I/are they going to get better?

Sometimes the young people and their families are looking for a prognosis: this is an important question and an opportunity for instilling hope.

There is no point in being unreasonably optimistic or cheerful – some families may find this disrespectful and may feel you did not understand their problems. The question also implies that you are seen as an expert and that you have experience and access to an evidence base.

It is essential to provide evidence to support your statements – the best evidence to support your statement is a combination of research findings applied to the young person's circumstances.

One way to respond could be:

Key answer

On the basis of our discussion it appears that there are the following factors (name them) that apply to your family/to the young person. Research shows that they are associated with positive outcomes.

1. Resilience/positive prognostic factors in young people:
   - problem-solving abilities
   - social skills
   - contact with at least one supportive carer
   - successful experience at school
   - good self-esteem
   - ability to adapt to changes
   - having an internal locus of control.
2. Family resilience/positive prognostic factors:
   - open lines of communication
   - commitment to one another
   - showing appreciation for one another
   - dealing with crises in a positive way
   - spiritual wellness.

Assessment Manual

3. Environmental resilience/positive prognostic factors:
   - at least one good friend/supportive adult
   - attending a good school
   - attending clubs and interest groups
   - being in touch with the local community.

Further instilling of hope

Key question

Tell me three things you are good at.

Tell me three things your daughter is good at/you like about your daughter.

You can further develop these questions based on Aaron Beck's 'hope box exercise'. Adjust your further questions depending on the answers to the key question.

Explore the things that the young person:

achieved in the past (school, sports, music, work experience);

enjoyed in the past (family trips, holidays, birthday celebrations)

likes now;

may achieve in the future (profession, skill, relationships);

might enjoy in the future or is looking forward to;

finally, explore the people *whose company they enjoy.*

If the young person finds this difficult, introduce the formulation:

> *If things were to improve, what might you find yourself doing/looking forward to in the future?*

Warning: If you cannot establish any of the above positive prognostic factors, you should seriously consider:

1. whether the young person is depressed;
2. whether the young person is safe to be discharged home;
3. whether there is a high risk of further self-harm or suicide.

> *In summary, the instillation of hope is a subtle process that requires attention to and highlighting of any positive predictive factors, the ability to co-construct a better future and the ability to set goals and targets. The role of the therapist is of paramount importance and is based on the therapist's professional knowledge, attention to detail and optimism.*

CHAPTER 14

ASSESSING AND ENHANCING MOTIVATION

Dennis Ougrin

Assessing and enhancing motivation

This chapter is structured in the following way. First, a brief discussion of the principles of exploring and enhancing motivation is proposed. Then there is an algorithm of a motivational intervention applied to a young person presenting with self-harm. The chapter is concluded with a real-life example of using motivational skills to engage a young person.

Motivational interviewing (MI) was originally used for patients with substance misuse problems; however there is more and more evidence for other applications of motivational principles in different areas. The aim of this chapter is not to describe the pure MI process. The authors will try to use MI ideas to explore and enhance young people's motivation to create 'exits' from the diagram.

Basically, MI principles could be applied to any target in the diagram that the young person is in two minds about. For example, this could be self-harm itself, or using drugs, or skiving from school or even unprotected sex.

You may be faced with an apparent motivation problem if a young person refuses to engage with your assessment. An example at the end of this chapter explores motivational work under these circumstances. It is likely that people with poor motivation may also be hopeless and angry – they may refuse to engage with you and may want to leave the assessment before speaking to you. They may have been rude to other professionals, particularly if they felt patronised or criticised (remember reciprocal roles?). They may refuse to answer any questions, especially the ones everyone is particularly keen on, like do you still want to die?

Before setting out to assess and enhance motivation, it is important to bear in mind the following:

- Motivation is a spectrum and it is very rare to have 0 per cent or 100 per cent level of motivation to do anything.
- Motivation varies over time. Acute crisis provides an opportunity to review the level of motivation and may be associated with enhanced or decreased motivation to change.

Assessment Manual

- Motivation could be specific – young people might have very different motivation for different targets; for example, motivation to stop self-harm might be great, whereas motivation to stop smoking cannabis might be low or vice versa.
- Motivation is interpersonal. The assumption should be that the young person has resources and capacity to change. Using a collaborative approach, avoiding confrontation and respecting the young person's autonomy is likely to bring these resources to the fore.

Let's revisit the cycle of change, a concept most mental health professionals will be familiar with (Figure 14.1).

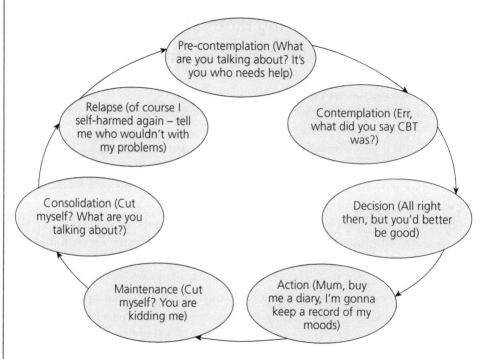

Figure 14.1 The cycle of change.

Usually it is obvious where the young person is in this cycle – in practice when assessing young people presenting with self-harm, the therapists are frequently faced with ambivalence. No matter where the young person is on the cycle of change, or what the target problem is, the following MI principles apply:

1. Expressing empathy – accepting the young person's point of view without necessarily approving or disapproving. Reflection is the best way to show this.
2. Developing discrepancy – highlighting the difference between the way things are now and the way the young person prefers them to be. Eliciting change talk and weighing pros and cons are tools used to develop discrepancy.

3. Supporting self-efficacy – belief that the young person has the necessary resources to affect change. Tools for supporting self-efficacy are using the change rulers and exploring the young person's successes in the past.
4. Rolling with resistance – if you sense resistance, e.g. 'I dunno' replies, anger or yawning – get away from it and change strategy. Avoid arguments – if you find yourself joining in with an argument stop and reflect – did you enter into the critical/omnipotent reciprocal role? Can you acknowledge this?

If you sense resistance it may be a signal to change tactics. The young person might need a break or it may be useful to engage the significant others to help the young person feel more relaxed. Perhaps you need to select another TA tool from the manual.

Before you consider these options, the following immediate responses have been advocated:

- Empathic reflection – comment on the feeling/perception/idea behind the statement (e.g. 'You seem angry with the way things have gone for you today'; 'It must be very frustrating to wait for four hours in the emergency department' (ED); 'It seems you think no one is able to understand you').
- Amplified reflection – reflect back the young person's statement with exaggeration, e.g. Young Person (YP): 'Most of my friends smoke cannabis.' Therapist (T): 'So if you stopped smoking you would have no friends left'. This usually helps the young person realise the evidence to the contrary of your suggestion.
- Double-sided reflection – reflect back both the negatives and the positives. T: 'You feel frustrated with the long wait *and* you decided to stay until I arrive'.
- Reframing YP: 'My mother is constantly nagging me to stop cutting'. T: 'It seems your mother is very concerned about your cutting'.
- Make an open question/statement – YP: refuses to speak T: 'I am wondering what you might be experiencing right now?'
- Move to a different topic – T: 'I can see that talking about self-harm is difficult for you right now *and* I would really like to understand you better. Perhaps you could tell me what you like doing after school?' Again note the use of *and* rather then *but*. This ensures the young person's feelings are not invalidated.

The OARS could provide a communication framework or the non-directive components of MI. OARS stands for:

- Open-ended questions
- Affirming strengths and change efforts
- Reflective statements
- Summaries.

Assessment Manual

Open-ended questions

Open-ended questions require more than yes/no answers:

- How will you know this assessment was useful?
- Tell me a little about yourself?
- In what way does self-harm affect your life?

Open-ended questions is a general umbrella term and asking open questions is only part of the 'O' in OARS.

In broader sense it is also about an open approach to the young person. Remember game theory, originally devised in economics by von Neumann and Morgenstern – people are more likely to be open and fair with you if they think you are open and fair with them. When approaching a young person, be polite and open about yourself – tell them your occupation and the purpose of the assessment. Tell them about your work and yourself (as much as feels comfortable and maintains professional boundaries) – this is likely to improve engagement.

Affirmation

This is about expressing confidence in the young person's ability to achieve the targets:

- You seem to have done a lot of thinking about the cannabis use already
- It sounds like you were reluctant to see me and you decided to stay (note the use of 'and' instead of 'but').

Affirmation could be difficult to do for some therapists, but there is always something to highlight as a positive in a young person. Acknowledge that the young person has not left and is still talking to you. Do not lie, however – young people are very sensitive to false statements without evidence. Note when the young person was honest, open, considerate etc.

Reflection

Reflective statements clarify and capture the young person's meaning

So, you used to think that cutting was a good way of dealing with your anger, and now you feel it interferes with your relationships.

You could simply repeat what the young person tells you, but a better way to reflect is to rephrase or paraphrase:

Young person: My dad always tells me to get lost when I need his help. It always makes me feel angry and I smoke cannabis, but now that makes me feel even worse.

Assessment Manual

Therapist: It sounds like you find it difficult to cope with rejection and that drugs don't help you deal with anger anymore.

Reflect the young person's feelings – do they seem angry, upset, exasperated. Express empathy – you need to show that the young person's feelings are understandable an interest in the young person's values, beliefs and feelings. You need to understand what the young person will be loosing by making a change.

Reflect the young person's meaning – comment on how important you felt their views were and what beliefs they might reflect.

One special type of summary frequently used in motivational work is the summary of both aspects of ambivalence – the main points of what the young person finds good and not so good about the behaviour they might like to change.

Summaries

Summaries highlight the main points the young person made.

> *Let me see if I understood you correctly. The main reasons why you are considering starting counselling is because you feel you could do with support after what you've been through, your friend felt better after her counselling sessions and you need to have someone who can listen to you.*

When doing motivation work at least some summaries are required – to check if you have understood and to highlight major points discussed. A therapeutic letter is of course one way to summarise the main aspects of the session.

The following five techniques constitute the directive elements of motivational work: exploring ambivalence, change rulers, evocative questions, strengthening commitment and planning change. The basic assumption is that the more the young person becomes aware of the reasons for change, the more they appreciate their own strength, resources and ability, the more likely change becomes. OARS (the non-directive elements) are used alongside the directive techniques.

Exploring ambivalence

The motivational work in MI usually starts with exploring ambivalence:

Key question

What is good about the (target behaviour, e.g. self-harm, smoking cannabis)? What is not so good about it?

You can further develop this in the following ways:

1. Explore the impact of the target behaviour

Assessment Manual

> *How does the (target behaviour) affect you?*
> *How does the (target behaviour) affect other people?*
> *How does the (target behaviour) affect your relationships?*
> *What are the immediate consequences of the (target behaviour)?*
> *What are the long-term consequences of the (target behaviour)?*

2. Introduce the future perspectives.

> *If you had stopped the (target behaviour) how life would be different now*
> *If you stopped the (target behaviour) how life would be different in the future*
> *If you don't make any changes, what do you think will happen?*
> *Where would you like to be in a year from now? What do you hope would be different? How does (target behaviour) fit into this?*

3. Introduce other people's perspectives.

> *What do other people think about the (target behaviour)?*
> *If your (important other) were here what would they say?*
> *Who would be least surprised if you stopped the (target behaviour)?*
> *What would they notice?*

Summarise the ambivalence. Consider using a decision balance sheet (Figure 14.2).

Positive things about my self-harm for me <u>now</u>	Negative things about my self-harm for me <u>now</u>
Positive things about my self-harm in relation to others <u>now</u>	Negative things about my self-harm in relation to others <u>now</u>
Positive things about my self-harm <u>in the future</u>	Negative things about my self-harm <u>in the future</u>

Figure 14.2 A decision balance sheet.

Creating scales (change rulers)

Key question

On a scale of 0–10, with 0 having no motivation to change and 10 being ready to start changing things, where are you right now?

Having obtained a summary score for the overall motivation you can develop this part by exploring different elements of motivation.

Importance of change

How important is it that you change your target behaviour?

Not at all important									Very important	
0	1	2	3	4	5	6	7	8	9	10

Confidence to change

How confident are you that you can change your target behaviour?

Not at all confident									Very confident	
0	1	2	3	4	5	6	7	8	9	10

Readiness to change

How ready are you to change your target behaviour?

Not at all ready									Very ready	
0	1	2	3	4	5	6	7	8	9	10

Enhancing motivation: eliciting change talk (evocative questions)

Key question

How come your score is not zero – tell me more about it. Why else?
What would need to happen for you to move up one point?
You can develop this further by:

1. Introducing other people's perspective:

> *Who would be the most useful person to help you move up one point?*
> *Who else thinks that you should move up the scale? What are their arguments?*

2. Introducing the future perspective:

> *If you decided to move up the scale how would you do it?*
> *Why would you want to increase your motivation?*
> *If you don't make any changes, what do you think will happen?*
> *Where would you like your motivation to be in the future?*

3. Introducing the young person's skills and strengths:

> *What strengths could you draw on to move up the scale?*
> *In what ways would it be good for you to move up the scale?*

4. Other evocative questions:

- Can you tell me about the time before (the target problem behaviour)? What was it like?
- What may happen if things continue as they are?
- If you stop (the target problem behaviour) how would your life be different?
- What would your life be like in 1 year's time?
- What is the worst that can happen if you don't change?
- What is the best that can happen if you do change?
- How does (the target problem behaviour) fit with what you want to do in the future (e.g. going to college, having a boyfriend, travelling abroad)?

Finally, it is possible that the young person could be ready to plan change. Before you move to the phase of planning change you need to summarise the information elicited: the pros and cons of change, where the young person is on the rulers of change, the impact of the problem and reasons for change. It is likely that the young person is high on the measures of readiness, ability and confidence to change before this stage is reached. The framework below could be helpful to follow from this point.

Key question

It sounds like you are ready to change things – what do you think would be the best way to do it?

The worksheet in Figure 14.3 may help the young person structure their thoughts.

So, in summary the algorithm for using motivational work is as follows:

1. Identify target
2. Explore/enhance ambivalence
3. Elicit change talk

4. explore components of motivation to change
5. prepare a plan.

The changes I want to make (or continue making) are:
The most important reasons why I want to make these changes are:
The steps I plan to take in changing are:
The ways other people can help me, and how I can ask for their support:
I will know my plan is working if:
Some things that could interfere with my plan are:
What I will do if the plan isn't working:

Figure 14.3 Change plan worksheet.

Assessment Manual

Please note that it is highly unlikely that a young person is going to go through the whole of the algorithm. It is not only unlikely but also undesirable to drag the young person along. Remember to stay with your client and provide a scaffolding rather then playing tug of war.

Example of Nadia

A 17-year-old White British young lady presented following an overdose of Dihydrocodeine tablets (that belonged to her mother who is suffering from cancer) with the background of a deterioration in her relationships with her mother and pressures at college.

The assessing psychiatric liaison nurse (PLN) and ED nurses formed a very unfavourable view of Nadia as she reportedly acted in an aggressive and abusive way. She refused to be assessed by the PLN stating that she felt patronised. When the assessing clinician entered the ED Nadia was packing her belongings ready to go home without entering into any further discussions. The exchange in Table 14.1 then took place.

Table 14.1 Exchange between Nadia and therapist

Therapist	Nadia	Therapist's thoughts
[smiling, open gestures] Hello, Nadia, my name is Dennis. I work for the department of psychological medicine	Continues packing	Not even eye contact – she must be fuming. It would be a shame to call security to keep her in, but might have to resort to this as she isn't even medically cleared
[sitting down at the edge of her cubicle area, without invading her territory] you seem quite upset and perhaps angry (reflection)	You bet I'm upset. Everybody has been so fucking nasty and patronising, especially that fat bitch	Is she referring to the PLN? Staff abuse can't be tolerated, but is now a good time to set boundaries?
I think I would feel the same if I were you – seems you've been through tough times [empathic comment]	Yeah, what do you know about tough times, you do this for money and you don't give a shit about me	She is rejecting/criticising me – there's your reciprocal role. Anyway, let's see how she would respond to a bit of openness and humour
Well the money isn't as good as in second-hand car sales [trying to deflect resistance with humour]. I work mainly with three groups of people (open statement, self-disclosure)	Yeah? [stopped packing]	OK, let's go
I work with some young people who have serious psychiatric illness [she rolled her eyes up]. They are a small group. Most young people are the ones who do not fulfil their potential, usually for reasons that are not very clear to begin with. I try to help them do better and succeed in whatever it is that they want to do [another open statement, self-disclosure]	You said there were three groups	I know this – you look more interested than I thought you might – is achieving important to you?
Yes, the third small group are the young people who are very gifted but need extra help to use their talent	Ah – that's not gonna be me. Anyway, you are the only polite person in this place	Oh-oh, you are not trying to idealise me? You might not like some of the things I say later on. Splitting, don't forget about splitting.

PLN, psychiatric liaison nurse.

And so the rest of the history is abbreviated here.

Nadia felt miserable after several arguments with her mother. This was triggered by her mother criticising Nadia for not doing well at college and for not being interested in her future. The background is of frequent arguments, pressure to perform from family and not being able to match the family expectations. This is particularly problematic due to unfavourable comparisons with her cousin who is doing very well and is studying medicine. Mother suffered from bouts of depression and Nadia often felt unloved and had to be looked after by an aunt.

After the index argument, Nadia felt unable to cope, confused and wanted it all to go away. She took an overdose that was not premeditated and she seemed confused about her intent.

There is an extensive history of depressive symptoms and worsening of cannabis misuse that preceded depression. There was significant deterioration in Nadia's college performance and she has not been in touch with her friends as much, having started to use cannabis on her own. Nadia admitted to having images of jumping out of the window of her flat, but she is always able to reason that the images are just that and there are people who might get upset if she hurt herself. The presentation was in the context of imminent college exams.

Her mother was present during the assessment, but Nadia did not feel comfortable being assessed in her mother's presence but agreed for the therapist to interview mother separately.

Nadia's diagram is shown in Figure 14.4.

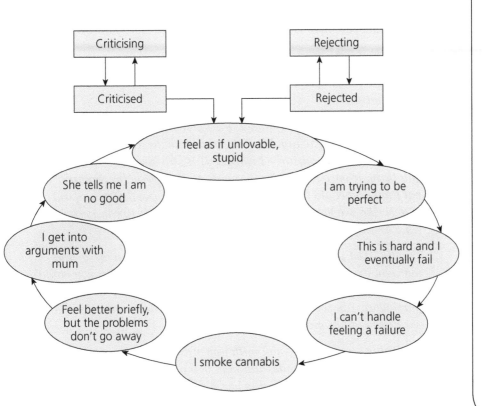

Figure 14.4 Nadia's diagram.

As you will see from the diagram, there are several potential targets for exploring exits, however, we focused on the role cannabis played in the vicious cycle. This is the summary of the discussion using the techniques described above.

Cannabis has several important functions in Nadia's life. It dampens her feelings allows her to stay in touch with some of the friends and makes her more social. On the other hand, the amount of cannabis she used has increased dramatically, costing her as much as $50 a week and making her borrow money. She also lost many friends, especially the ones she thought would disapprove of her cannabis use. Although she felt better in the short term, cannabis did not take her problems away. She was quite scared of what her mother would do if she found out about the extent of her cannabis problem. Of note, Nadia did not believe cannabis had any undesirable effects on her health, although she had quite a lot of drug education at school. Cannabis use did not particularly fit with her future plans. She wanted to save money and thought being in debt was not good.

On balance, Nadia thought it would be a good idea to stop using cannabis. Her motivation to stop was rated as 8 out of 10 (composite). She rated herself particularly high on importance (10/10), but lower on readiness (6/10). Nadia wasn't sure what would increase her readiness, but on reflection thought her uncle (who had a drug problem but stopped using drugs) might be worth talking to. She wanted to ring the young persons' drug and alcohol service for more information.

Understanding Letter

Dear Nadia

As promised, I am sending you this letter following our discussion earlier today. You will recognise the diagram above that you helped me draw – I wonder if it still looks right, or do you think it may need to be changed. As you know the diagram is not final and could be changed as there are many different ways to describe people's behaviour. Plus it will definitely change over time and will need re-thinking.

I really liked your idea that the diagram looked like a circle and that you could break it in more then one place. Although you could think of a few possible targets in the diagram, one stood out in particular. You seemed in two minds about using cannabis and wanted to talk some more about it.

Cannabis seems to help you with anger and you enjoy smoking with some of your friends, although you also have friends with strong views against cannabis use. Cannabis also seems to help you be funny and make friends more easily.

There are also other things that are not so good about smoking cannabis. You seemed particularly worried that you needed to smoke more and more and seem not to get stoned as easily as before. Smoking costs you as much as £50 a week and you were worried that you would not be able to repay the people you borrowed the money from. I thought more about this after the assessment and wondered if I understood how much of a problem this is for you. I know that you owe about £100 now. If you are more worried about it than I thought, you are welcome to call me any time before we meet again next Wednesday.

You also thought that the reason why Richard and Daljit did not come to your birthday was because they did not want to be with people who smoked dope and you were worried it may be difficult to keep their friendship. You also told me that even though you felt better when you smoked cannabis the problems were always there in the morning – if anything it was more difficult to deal with them if you kept putting them off. Finally you thought your mum could stop giving you pocket money and could scream and shout at you if she found out how much cannabis you smoked.

I know that you want to become a beautician and that you thought smoking cannabis is not going to help you with that. You were worried you would have to give up studying and get a full-time job to be able to pay for it and to settle your debts.

You thought giving up smoking was very important but you were not quite ready to do it. You rated your readiness as 6 out of 10 and thought you might see your uncle Marinos over the weekend who might understand you better and might give you some good advice. Do you think he would agree to come to our next session on Wednesday? Do you think this would be helpful?

You wanted to ring Ask Frank to find out more about cannabis – here is the number again. I would be happy to answer any questions about the effects of cannabis if these are still unclear and if I know the answers – maybe I should look it up before our next meeting.

Dennis

In summary, assessing and enhancing young people's motivation to change is a complex phenomenon that is problem-specific and may vary considerably over time. The young person's position on the cycle of change will determine the most profitable intervention. Motivation work may inform the work on identifying potential exits from the diagrams.

Reference

1.   Rollnick S, Miller WR. *Motivational interviewing: preparing people for change*, 2nd edition. New York, NY: Guildford Press 2002.

Assessment Manual

CHAPTER 15

USING A FUTURE-ORIENTED REFLEXIVE APPROACH

Dennis Ougrin

Introduction

This approach is derived from solution-focused, narrative and systemic traditions and could potentially be applied to any point in the diagram. It is best to ask the young person (and a carer if available) which part of the diagram is ideally worth targeting – it may be worth formulating a target problem before engaging in future-oriented reflexive questioning. An informant is particularly valuable in this approach – you will see that they can be an invaluable resource if the young person gets stuck or needs encouragement. The general algorithm of the session is based on the following questions:

1. Opening: ask both the young person and the carer(s)

Key question

What are your greatest hopes for this assessment?
Other openings:

- How would you know if this assessment had been useful after we've finished?
- What would need to happen so that on your way home from here you tell yourself 'That assessment was useful'?
- What would (your important other) hope will be different as a result of this assessment?

2. Constructing preferred future

Key question

Imagine your problem is no longer bothering you – how would you know this was the case?
Try to explore the answers in detail – ask about specific examples and people involved. Explore how things would be different in:

1. the way the young person would behave, feel, think and act at home, at school and at leisure;
2. the way that other people would behave, feel, think and act in response;
3. the way the relationship with other people would be different – family, friends, teachers etc. Ask what family members might do to make the relationships work better.

Note: the preferred future has to be kept positive. Use 'instead questions' to reframe the preferred future. For example:

Young person: I wish my mother wouldn't argue with me
   Therapist: What would you prefer your mother did instead?

Equally the danger might be to channel negative emotions into someone who is not present.

   Mother: I wish my husband would spend more time with the family
Therapist: Even if your husband does not spend more time with the family, how would you know things were better regardless?

> *What would need to happen for your husband to spend more time with the family?*

If the preferred future is unrealistic, ask:

How would [never going to school again] be good for you?
Would you like to achieve that and go to school?

Consider the miracle question

Suppose you were to go home after this assessment, do whatever you usually do for the rest of the day and then go to sleep. But while you were asleep a miracle happened and the [target problem or all problems] were solved. When you wake up tomorrow, how would [both of] you be able to tell?

Remember that the miracle question is a strong remedy and some young people/families may not be ready for it.

Consider these solution-focused questions for the family who are less optimistic:

> *Imagine your problem got a little bit better. How would you know that?*
> *What are you doing that keeps you going and stops you giving up?*
> *What are you doing that prevents things from getting even worse?*

Younger adolescents

Consider the following approach for the families/young people who may find abstract construction of the preferred future difficult. Tie the change to specific daily activities starting first thing in the morning:

> *Suppose the [target problem] resolved/improved overnight – what would be the first thing in the morning that would be different? What else?*
>
> *What would be different when you got to school? During the first lesson? During the break? When you got home after school?*

Take the young person through a typical day, noticing all changes that would go with an improvement of the target problem.

Introduce another person's perspective

> *Who would be the most likely person to notice [the target problem] was getting better?*
>
> *How will (the important other) know that things are getting better?*
>
> *What will be the first thing they will notice? What next?*

Introduce the idea of resources

> *Who/what might be helpful in getting the target problem resolved? What strengths/qualities would you use to achieve this? What difference will this make to you in the future?*

In general, the therapist must use their judgement to decide on the 'strengths' of the questions used – a little like the decision to use fluoxetine, duloxetine or a combination of venlafaxine and mirtazapine for depression. The more pessimistic the young person and family are the more unassuming the questions should be (Table 15.1).

3. Constructing a scale – bridging the elements of the preferred future that already exist

Key question

On a scale of 0–10, 0 being the worst that the [target problem] has been in your life and 10 being the achievement of your greatest hopes, where are you now? This could be developed further:

Table 15.1 Examples of questions

Optimistic		Strong
	How would you know/imagine that a miracle happened and that all of the problems have resolved?	
	How would you know/Imagine this problem is no longer bothering you?	
	How would you know/Imagine this problem got a little better?	
	Suppose things did not change very much in the next few days, what would be the first little thing that would tell you things are getting better?	
	What are you doing that keeps you going and stops you giving up?	
	What are you doing that prevents things from getting even worse?	
Pessimistic		Weak

What is it that you are doing that means you are at (point on scale) and not 0

Where on the scale represents good enough for you?

What will you be doing that will tell you that you have moved up one point?

If still 0 now, how would you know if you moved up a point?

What do you think is the most likely thing that will change in the next week

How would [the important person] know you have moved up one point

What strengths would you use to go up a point?

Consider asking how come things are not even worse, especially if the young person seems very pessimistic.

Other scales are discussed below.

Confidence scale

How confident are you that you can achieve your 'good enough' point?

Not at all confident   Very confident

| 0 | 1 | 2 | 3 | 4 | 5 | 6 | 7 | 8 | 9 | 10 |

Safety scale

On a scale 0 to 10, with 0 representing you knowing that you can't keep yourself safe and 10 knowing for certain that you will be safe, where do you see yourself on this scale?

Not at all safe   Very safe?

0	1	2	3	4	5	6	7	8	9	10

4. Elements of preferred future that already exist.

Key question

Thank you for sharing your preferred future with me. It sounds quite realistic. How much of it is already happening?

> *What/who helps you to achieve this?*
> *What was different about last weekend – what did you do?*
> *What does it say about you?*
> *When you faced this problem in the past how did you resolve it?*
> *What might your (important person) like about the way you dealt with it?*
> *When in the last few days/weeks have you seen something, even in a small way of what you are hoping to see in the future?*

Review your history – is there any other evidence of elements of the preferred future. Explore these in detail. For example, part of the preferred future might be that the young person does their homework regularly. You also know that the young person was doing their homework yesterday from your history.

How come the young person was doing her homework?
What was different?
What/who helped?
What does it say about the young person?

> *Ask a carer: Bearing this in mind, what does it say to you about their personality/the kind of person he/she is?*

5. Exceptions

Key question

When doesn't the target problem happen?
This could be developed further:

> *When doesn't the target problem last as long?*
> *When is it less in charge?*
> *When are the times that you feel better?*
> *When do you resist the urge to (self-harm)?*
> *What/who helps you to be in charge of the target problem?*
> *What does it say about you/ your character/ your strengths?*
> *What did it take to achieve it?*

6. Tasks for the next few days (optional)

1. I (or one of my colleagues) will see you in the next seven days. When we next meet, you might like to tell me what changes you have noticed
2. What you might like to do in the next few days is to pay attention to the times when your [target problem] is not bothering you. You might like to tell me (or the person offering follow up) what you noticed
3. What you might like to do in the next few days is to pay attention to the times when things are the way you'd like them to be/ when you feel better. You might like to tell me (the person offering follow up) what you noticed and what/who helped.

7. Summary of the session highlighting strengths

1. Use the young person's language
2. Do not overwhelm the young person with material
3. Check if you got it right.

Case example

The following is a brief history and a diagram for Gabriella. She is a 13-year-old young lady of White British/Caribbean ancestry presenting with self-harm, on and off, since the age of 12 years, daily cannabis use and concerns that she was a member of a gang. Her parents have been having significant marital problems. Her father, a strict disciplinarian, was expecting Gabriella to obey his instructions at all times, not to use any substances, to be at home by 7 pm every day and to stop seeing all of her current friends as they were a negative influence on her. He was also insisting on going through Gabriella's belongings and mobile phone address book and insisting on checking if she had her periods for fears of her becoming pregnant.

Gabriella's mother was suffering from depression and had little input into Gabriella's upbringing during periods of illness, although when she was well she was much more involved. She generally sided with Gabriella, perceiving the father's strict parenting style as the root of the problem but also felt unable to care for Gabriella at various points in her life.

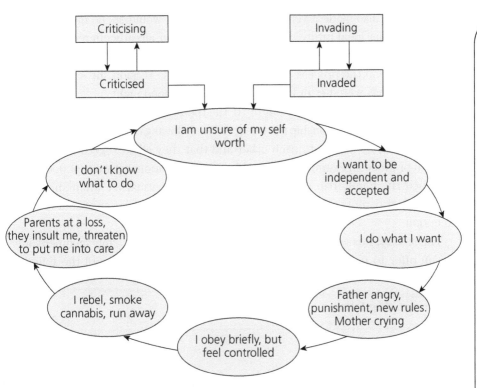

Figure 15.1 Gabriella's diagram.

The immediate precipitant to the presentation was a break-up with a boyfriend and an increase in self-harming behaviour (Figure 15.1).

The target problem here was designated as the difficult relationship between Gabriella and her parents, especially the father. When asked how the family would know if this was a worthwhile session, father immediately stated that the only way forward is for Gabriella to do as she is told and that he will not compromise under any circumstances. Gabriella and her mother said that they would value an opportunity to have their views heard. After some debate (and compromise) the current relationship between parents and Gabriella was rated as 1 out of 10. Each member of the family was asked how they would know that things have moved up one point to 2 out of 10. When mutual demands and accusations surfaced, the question was rephrased to what each family member would do to contribute to this. The main agent of change (somewhat surprisingly) appeared to be the father. When asked what the family would do instead of engaging in power struggles he offered a variety of activities that all family members would enjoy. Gabriella then suggested that she would aim to stay at home more often (mother encouraged her with a surprised/happy remark) and listed several other things she could do before saying, 'Hang on this wouldn't be 2 out of 10, this would be 7 out of 10 already' (everyone

Assessment Manual

laughed). She also made it very clear that her father would spend more time with the family in her ideal future. In some ways the father already offered the same in his opening remarks. Mother was saying very little and the therapist was worried about her role in the process. Towards the end of the session she said she would know that things were better if she kissed Gabriella good night.

Going back to the rating of 1 out of 10, the therapist explored what factors were responsible for the relationship not being 0. The following contributions were made: the fact that they all talk to each other and that they all sit together now. When asked to produce an example that would show the relationship was not 0, Gabriella described the family trip to a large out-of-town supermarket when she walked alongside her parents and shared a joke with her father – this was of course also an exception.

The session was concluded with a plan derived from the family members' ideas and an offer to notice the elements of the preferred future until the follow-up session.

Understanding Letter

Hi Gabby,

First of all, I wanted to thank you for sharing so much of your life story with me and also to thank your parents for being open about the family difficulties.

I enclose the diagram that we made. It mainly describes your relationship with your parents and I'm sure there are many other things that could be in the diagram but are not – as you know we could change it and rethink it as we continue to work.

In this letter I thought I should briefly recap the main ideas that you and your parents discussed – would you feel comfortable sharing this letter with your parents? If not, I could write a separate letter to them or we could even write one together.

As you may remember, the relationship between the family members was rated as 1 out of 10. I was wondering if this rating was still true at the end of the session but forgot to ask you. What did you think?

I wanted to check with you if I forgot anything important that all of you mentioned about how you would know things were getting better. Your father thought of loads of things that you have enjoyed in the past, like going to the Tate Modern, going on a cycling trip in Norfolk and going to visit his brother who is a musician and whom I thought you liked very much. It seems you were particularly keen on the visit to your uncle Barry. I wonder what uncle Barry would have said had he been sitting in the session.

You thought that if you stayed at home more often and did your schoolwork, and did your bed in the morning, then this would contribute to a better relationship in the family, although that would definitely be more than 2 out of 10. You also thought that sharing jokes, having a meal together and spending time together would be part of this future change. I was very impressed with your observation that you and your parents were together at the assessment and that you did make an effort to do your homework and how that made a difference at school. The shopping trip to Bluewater particularly impressed me. You mentioned that you joked about your father being a shopaholic and how you even held hands there briefly. I thought it was important that you and your parents felt comfortable talking about your feelings of warmth towards each other.

Your mum then also mentioned that she would know things were getting better if you had a good night kiss – this used to happen a lot in the past and used to make her feel good.

Gabby, as you know, I will see you next week and if you have an opportunity I would be interested to know if you (or your parents) can notice any more examples of an improving relationship over the next few days.

With best regards

Dennis

In summary, future-oriented reflexive questions are a powerful tool in TA. They usually draw on the family strengths and provide a framework for change. They could be targeted towards a specific problem or a more general issue as in the example above. The work could be done with young people with or without other family members. These questions can usually provide a benign and positive atmosphere except perhaps in the most hopeless individuals.

CHAPTER 16

PROBLEM-SOLVING TECHNIQUES

Audrey V. Ng

Problem solving

A problem-solving approach could be applied at several points in the procedural sequence. Using a problem-solving approach might be particularly helpful in creating exits from the diagram at the points where the young person feels stuck.

It is important to try and understand the magnitude of the problem(s) that the young person is experiencing. Get as complete a picture as possible so that the young person knows that you can appreciate what they are going through otherwise you will invariably be greeted with the response 'you don't understand' however empathetic you are. Aim to convey that if the problems are broken into sections it is often possible to find a solution that can be implemented successfully.

The basic algorithm of a problem-solving approach is very simple:

1. What is my problem (define)
2. What are the possible solutions (brainstorm and write them down)
3. What are the consequences (evaluate short- and long-term consequences)
4. Choose one solution
5. Implement
6. Evaluate outcome, learn from mistakes
7. Modify solution, reapply solution.

Before looking at this in more detail, let's consider the example of Patrick.

Example of Patrick

Patrick is a 12-year-old boy of Black British origin. He presented to a community team following an urgent referral via his GP. During a routine GP appointment he broke down in tears when the GP commented on his weight. He then stated that he could no longer stand bullying and that he tried to hang himself recently. He did not feel any regret for the attempted hanging and confessed to thinking about 'ending it all' at least weekly. The reason why he was still alive was that his mum would be upset if he died.

The history is as follows. Patrick is the youngest child in the family and he has adult half-siblings on both his mother's and his father's side. His parents are of Caribbean origin and are both retired. Patrick's parents were quite guarded about the information they disclosed and checked several times that the assessment was confidential. Patrick did not come across as particularly verbal and his final diagram reflected the paucity of the information obtained.

There was little information available about Patrick's early life or the family relationships. The only area that the family were prepared to discuss in detail was the problem of bullying at school. This had been going on for about 12 months, since Patrick started his secondary school. He was called 'fat' and 'pig' as well as 'droplip', the latter referring to a gap between his lips. The bullying was fairly universal and he was particularly worried about the girls joining in with the boys. This made him feel bad. He was trying to ignore the bullying but would eventually blow up and would kick and swear at his abusers. This would then attract the teacher's attention and he gradually became very unpopular with the teachers. The teachers reported to parents that although Patrick was bullied he would also bully others. His school grades were in decline and he developed some depressive symptoms.

His parents did not know about the extent of the bullying and were certainly unaware of the impact it had on Patrick until the GP appointment.

Although very little information was presented, the diagram in Figure 16.1 was drawn with Patrick's help.

The session was built around problem solving.

Steps to helping the young person problem solve are listed below.

Step 1: Identify the problem

Key question

What is the problem that you are facing?

> *What would you like to change in your life?*
> *What would be your wish if you had a magic wand?*
> *How would you know things were getting better?*

Patrick was clear that bullying was the most pressing problem in his life.

Step 2: Brainstorm and generate solutions

Key question

I'd like you to imagine that everything is possible today. I'd like you to tell me what you think some of the ways of solving this problem might be?

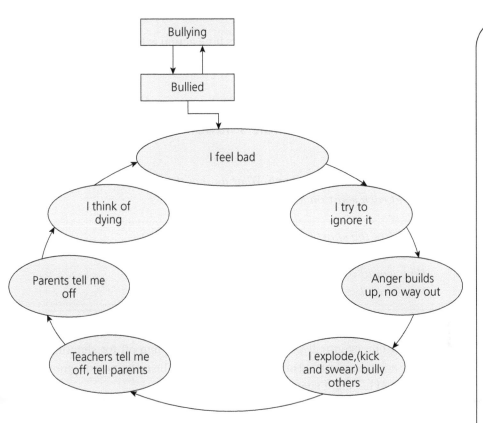

Figure 16.1 Patrick's diagram.

What would be the ideal solution?
What would be a good enough solution?
What has helped with the problem in the past?
If an important other was sitting in this chair next to me what would they say?
Imagine that a young person's hero were here what would they say the solution might be?
Let me ask your family now, can you add to this list?
What other solutions might help?

Patrick and his parents came up with the following solutions:

1. Never go to school again
2. Go to another school
3. Stand up to bullies
4. Ignore bullies

Assessment Manual

5. Tell the teachers about bullying
6. Parents to put pressure on teachers if no action is taken
7. Parents to speak with the parents of the bullies
8. Patrick to stop bullying other kids
9. Patrick to lose weight.

Step 3: Discuss each possible solution

Key question

Let's take the solution one by one. What do you think the good and not so good points about each solution are?

> *What are the short term consequences?*
> *What are the long-term consequences?*
> *How would it affect you?*
> *How would it affect other people?*

Patrick thought of ignoring the bullies: on the positive side it is likely they would stop bullying him eventually, teachers would not tell him off for shouting and he wouldn't be accused of ratting on fellow students. On the negative side ignoring may not be easy and he might snap eventually.

Step 4: Choose the best solution or even combination of solutions

Key question

Having gone through the options, what solution would you like to choose first?

> *What do you think is the most promising solution?*
> *What solution may be easiest to implement?*
> *What solution may be the quickest?*
> *What solution would (important other) pick?*
> *What solution would (the young person's hero) pick?*
> *What solution would the young person recommend to their best friend?*
> *Can you use a combination of two or more solutions?*
> *If you imagine yourself one year from now, which solution would you be most proud of choosing?*

Having discussed several most promising solutions, Patrick decided to try and ignore the bullies while at the same time stop bullying others.

Step 5: Plan how you are going to carry out the solution

Key question

Tell me in detail how are you going to carry out the solution?

> *What would be the first thing you will do?*
> *What will be next?*
> *What will be the most difficult thing about this solution?*
> *When may be the most difficult time?*
> *Who/what may help?*
> *Have you tried a similar solution before? What was the outcome? What was difficult/good about it? What might you do differently?*
> *Let us pretend I am the bully. What would I say? How would you respond?*

Step 6: Evaluate how it is going

Key question

I/one of my colleagues will see you in the next few days. Would you let me/them know how it went?

Step 7: Learn from mistakes, reapply new/modified solution

In summary, a problem-solving algorithm is easy to implement and may create a viable exit from the diagram. It could be applied to any part of the diagram and is particularly useful in young people who perceive themselves to be stuck with no options. The key is to generate and evaluate as many solutions as possible using imaginative perspectives.

CHAPTER 17

USING SYSTEMIC AND NARRATIVE APPROACHES TO CREATE EXITS

Tobias Zundel

Introduction

One of the most valuable ways of creating exits from therapeutic assessment (TA) diagrams is using a systemic–narrative approach. The first part of this chapter will give a brief theoretical underpinning of the systemic–narrative approach to exploring exits. The latter part will look at specific step-by-step algorithms of putting these ideas into practice.

Theoretical underpinning of a systemic–narrative approach

In clinical practice systemic–narrative approaches are used in work with families, groups and also individuals. In TA of self-harm the aim is to employ some of these principles during the time alone with the young person as well as during any wider discussions involving family, carers or even social workers.

In some ways the ethos of therapeutic assessment is very much in tune with the fundamental ideas that gave rise to systemic and later narrative approaches to psychotherapy. In 1987, the influential systemic therapist Karl Tomm[1] published the first of his three papers titled 'Interventive interviewing'. He writes: 'A clinical interview affords far more opportunities to act therapeutically than most therapists realise'. In many respects Tomm's papers were influenced by, and followed on from the original Milan systemic group's seminal publications on hypothesising, circularity and neutrality. They suggest these three offer an 'invitation to curiosity'.

- Curiosity can be considered as a very good starting point from which to gain insight as well as being a driving force towards engaging in a therapeutic process.
- Circularity or circular questioning assumes that difficulties can only be understood in the context of interactions between the people in a system (e.g. family) and therefore it is not useful to think about one person as having a problem and other people as being problem free.

- Neutrality almost speaks for itself and is clearly of great significance in any self-harm assessment as the young person will undoubtedly be very sensitive to feeling judged (remember the judging–judged reciprocal roles?). Neutrality means 'actively avoiding the acceptance of any one position as more correct than another'.
- Hypothesising is something that all clinicians are likely to do whether they are aware of it or not. The Milan group described the functional value of the hypothesis in the context of the clinical interview, as 'guaranteeing the activity of the therapist, which consists in the tracking of relational patterns'. They also state that: 'The hypothesis, as such, is neither true nor false, but rather, more or less useful.'[2]

Systemic approach

The basic idea of a systemic approach is that the problematic behaviour (target behaviour), such as self-harm, can only be understood in the context of a system (for example, family or a social group). The assumption is that different elements of the system influence each other and it is the interaction between them that creates the target behaviour. In a system, the relationships, behaviours and meanings are all linked in a circular fashion. Change in one element of the system (e.g. mother–father interaction) is therefore likely to cause change in other elements of the system (for example, the children's behaviour) and vice versa.

Circular questions

Circular questions arose from within the systemic tradition and they informed the later development of narrative ideas. Basically circular questions explore the relationship between behaviour, beliefs, relationships and time.

In general circular questions are good at:

- making connections between the meaning of important events;
- making connections between the present, future hopes and past stories;
- making sense of everyone's actions;
- showing how everyone is doing their best given all the circumstances.

For therapists they can:

- enable a view of respecting the client as the expert in their life;
- stimulate and keep the therapist's curiosity alive;
- facilitate creative use of the patient's language.

Several examples of circular questions are shown using the example of Sarah. Please do not feel put off by the complicated names of the various types of questions – all these questions do is explore the interactions between the family beliefs, behaviours and relationships and the way these change over time.

Example of Sarah

Sarah is a 14-year-old Black British girl who presented with an overdose of five paracetamol tablets to a community team after an urgent referral by her GP. She came for her first appointment accompanied by her mother and stepfather. The overdose happened in the context of increasing family disputes. Sarah described a pattern of doing 'inappropriate' things, being scared of mother's anger and punishment, lying to avoid these. The lies would then be discovered and Sarah would feel angry with herself and guilty and frequently found herself thinking of self-harm.

Other stressors identified included daily arguments between her mother and sisters, overcrowding (three sisters sharing one bedroom) and the death of her maternal grandfather a month ago, who seems to have been a very important person for Sarah.

The immediate precipitant to the overdose was lying about using the computer (that she was already banned from using for earlier lying) and facing her mobile phone being taken away in the context of having been 'grounded' for the next three months because of previous lies.

Sarah's mother and father separated recently. Mother has a new partner whom Sarah has difficulties with. According to the mother's observation Sarah is trying very hard to 'test the boundaries' by making 'unreasonable requests' of her stepfather. Interestingly, she calls him 'father'.

Sarah's biological parents went through a violent spell in relation to which Sarah remembers feeling powerless and out of control. She feels guilty about not 'protecting' her mother.

Various types of circular questions could be used to explore this history further. **Sequential questions** enquire into interactional sequences of behaviour in specific circumstances, not in terms of feelings or interpretations.

> *When Sarah makes unreasonable demands of her step-father, what does her mother do?*

Action questions enquire into differences as indicated by behaviour rather than descriptions of individual characteristics. Descriptions such as: 'Sarah's impossible/disruptive' can be expanded.

> *What does she do that makes you describe her as disruptive?*

Classification (ranking) questions enquire into ranking of responses by family members to specific behaviour or specific interaction.

> *When you are feeling low who is most affected? Or who is best at cheering you up? Who next?*

Who notices most/first when you feel low?
Who do you think understands best what it is like to self-harm?
Who do you feel closest to when you feel like self-harming, who do you feel most distant from?

Diachronic questions (change before and after the problem) enquire into changes in behaviour that indicate a change in relationships at different points in time, before and after specific events.

Before you started self-harming, how did you use to cope with similar feelings when they arose?

Mind-reading questions (triadic questions, gossiping) examine the quality of communication in a family, showing the extent to which they are aware of each other's thoughts and feelings. These questions also reveal differences of opinion between family members. These questions are used to ask one member of the family about thoughts or feelings of another family member (or someone who is not present or deceased), or to comment on the relationship between two other family members.

(Asking the mother):What would your father have said about Sarah taking an overdose?
(Asking the stepfather): What could mum do differently to make Sarah feel less like self-harming?

Hypothetical questions enquire into differences of opinion with respect to imagined situations (past/current/future). Such questions release people from the concreteness of 'factual' answers and reveal hopes, fears and aspirations.

(Asking the stepfather) If Sarah left home to live with her father who do you think would be able to take her place for your partner?
If other people could see your thoughts and feelings, like looking in a crystal ball, who would be most interested/upset/helpful?

Future questions are used to encourage families to imagine the pattern of their relationships in future. These questions help them to gain a new position towards their own dilemmas.

If this situation continues for another year/5 years, what do you think will happen?

Assessment Manual (side margin text)

Narrative approach

The underlying concepts of narrative therapy and systemic therapy are in many ways related and in fact narrative therapy has largely grown out of the systemic tradition.

The basic idea of the narrative approach is that all people make sense of their life by creating stories. If a story is repeated many times it becomes dominant and in some ways it can determine the interactions in the system (for example a family).

Example of Sarah

Consider the case Sarah described above. She is caught in a vicious cycle of making mistakes, feeling anxious of the consequences, trying to cover up by telling lies, being punished disproportionately, leading to her breaking the rules of the punishment and so on. If we were to ask the family members what the young person was like, they could plausibly come up with a story along these lines. The young person makes loads of mistakes. She also gets scared and tends to lie to cover up for her mistakes. The underlying constructs are: the young person is rather stupid, a coward and a liar.

This story then acquires a life of its own. Everyone is expecting Sarah to lie, make mistakes and be scared of the consequences. Family are therefore more likely to notice this behaviour, confirming the dominant story. The times when the young person is creative, brave and honest may not get noticed or may be disregarded. In the end, the young person may start thinking about herself as being stupid, a coward and a liar and act accordingly.

These problematic or 'problem-saturated' narratives are often found in cases where young people self-harm. Both the patient and the parents regularly describe feeling stuck or trapped and being totally helpless with no way out. This can be interpreted as them following an overly restrictive script that they have 'learned by heart' and cannot break free from.

Finding and enriching non-dominant narratives

Despite dominant narratives being very powerful there always are other, weaker, peripheral narratives about the young person that could be found and made stronger. Sarah, for example may not only be a stupid, cowardly liar, but also a caring, creative artist. Finding and depicting these alternative narratives will represent exits from the diagram, often from the core pain. Two other tools are used in the narrative tradition to facilitate enrichment of the non-dominant narratives

Externalising behaviour

The strategy of externalising a target behaviour could be a very effective way of creating exits from the TA diagram. Externalising has three main functions:

1. Creating a distance between the young person and the target behaviour. For example, a therapist could externalise lying or self-harm by asking Sarah and her parents about the times when these target behaviours are prominent and the times when Sarah can control them.

2. Exploring the influence of the target problem on the young person, their relationships and beliefs over time. There is a fundamental emphasis on seeing problems in terms of how they manifest in relation to others and how they affect people's lives and relationships rather than as being located inside the person or defining who a person is.

3. Establishing what or who helps the target behaviour to be in control of the young person and conversely what or who helps the young person to be in control of the target behaviour.

Identifying unique outcomes (in the context of the externalised behaviour)

There is no target behaviour (for example self-harm) that is always in total control of the young person's life. Identifying unique outcomes means identifying the time when the target behaviour is absent or less prominent or the young person feels more of a sense of control over it.

A unique outcome is an occasion on which the established, typical cycle of events or narrative is disrupted in such a way that a different, ideally more positive or constructive, outcome arises. The TA diagram can be particularly helpful in pointing out the opportunities at which this can occur. Once such an example is identified, ideally by the patients themselves, this can be explored in detail to understand more about what was different on this occasion. In this way a young person may have an insight that enables them to feel less trapped and more empowered to influence events. It is also possible for the patient to start outlining what they would have to do in order to make such a unique outcome routine rather than unique.

White and Epston[3] wrote that when a unique outcome has been identified in a person's account of their influence in relation to the problem, this can 'facilitate performances of new meanings in the present, new meanings that enable persons to reach back and to revise their personal relationship histories'.

Applying systemic–narrative ideas to creating exits from a therapeutic assessment diagram

We will now describe the algorithms of using systemic–narrative approaches to creating exits from a diagram.

First, let's review the diagram created on the basis of the information gathered. The diagram showing Sarah's pattern of behaviour could be seen as the dominant (problem-saturated) narrative (Figure 17.1).

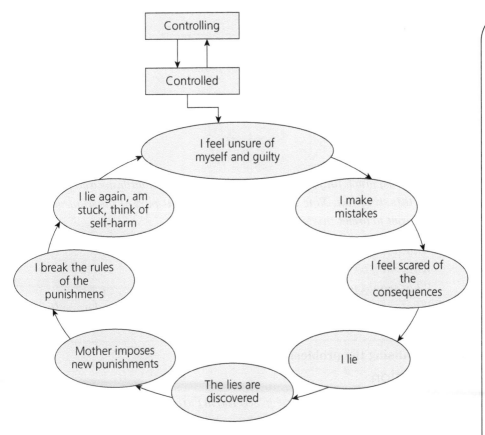

Figure 17.1 Sarah's diagram.

1. Opening: mapping the possible alternative narratives

Key question

What are your favourite activities?

> *What do you do well?*
>
> *What else?*
>
> *What are you good at?*
>
> *What do you like doing?*
>
> *What does it take to be able to do it so well?*
>
> *What does it say about you?*
>
> *If your best friend was sitting here what would they say about you*
>
> *What is your mum/dad good at?*
>
> *What would the view of a neutral outsider be?*

Asking parents:

> *Tell me three things that (the young person) is good at?*
> *What do you like about (the young person)?*
> *What is s/he good at?*
> *What does it say about (the young person)?*

2. Setting targets

Key question

Thank you very much for talking so much about yourself with me and for helping me draw this diagram. Now I'd like to ask you what part of the diagram could be your target to break this cycle?

> *What is the most important bit to change?*
> *What may be the easiest target?*
> *What would you like to change first?*
> *What would your (important other, e.g. mother) like to change first?*
> *How would this be good for you?*

3. Externalising the problem behaviour

Key question

How does the (target behaviour, e.g. self-harm) affect your life?

> *What/how should we name your problem?*
> *In what way does it make itself stronger/undermine you?*
> *Remember the times when you had more control over the problem, what was happening at those times?*
> *What kind of qualities does it highlight in you?*
> *What kind of person does it make you?*
> *How does it affect you?*
> *How would your life be different if you did more of (target behaviour)?*
> *How would your life be different if you did less of (target behaviour)?*
> *How does it affect your relationship with...?*
> *Who is most concerned/upset about (target behaviour)?*
> *Who is least upset about (target behaviour)?*
> *Who is most likely to be helpful?*
> *Who is least likely to be helpful?*
> *What would your (important other) say if s/he were sitting here?*
> *What do you think your (e.g. mum) would say if I asked her?*

Assessment Manual

What are your beliefs about (target behaviour)?
What is your theory on (target behaviour)?
I would like to know more about the (target behaviour).
What was your life like before (target behaviour) started
How did you used to cope before?
If we had this conversation one year ago/before the (target behaviour) started, what were you/your relationships like?
Imagine yourself in 5 years' time, what will you/your relationships target behaviour be like?

4. Looking for unique outcomes

Key question

Would it be OK if we now explore with you the times when this diagram does not work very well?

Have there been any times lately when (the target behaviour, e.g. self-harm) was lurking around and you stood up to it and did not allow it to push you around?
What did you tell yourself that helped you stand up to (target behaviour)?
What did you do?
What does it say about you?
How did other people help you be in control?
What else was happening at the same time?
In what way was it helpful?
Was there someone else there who helped you be in charge of (target behaviour)?
What would your (parents, grandparents or important others) say if they knew how you stood up to (target behaviour)?

5. Drawing exits onto the diagram

Key question

Do you mind if I write all of these things right here on the diagram?

6. Setting tasks for the next few days

Key question

I (one of my colleagues) will see you in the next few days. We would be very interested to learn more about the times between now and then when you were more in control of the target problem and how you managed to stand up to it.

Example of Sarah continued: the session

Sarah initially had troubles identifying what she was good at. Her mother helped out by saying Sarah was good at drawing and could be quite caring – the therapist asked mother to provide examples, which she duly did. Sarah's stepfather came up with his own observation that the parents could sometimes use Sarah as a messenger if they had a conflict with one of her sisters. He was happy to acknowledge that this highlights a very sensitive and diplomatic trait in Sarah.

Externalising lying was initially difficult but eventually all of the family started using the therapist's language of lying and Sarah as two separate entities. Lying was seen as a tricky enemy by everyone. Lying had powerful allies. The most powerful one was very long periods of punishment. In her fight with lying Sarah also had a powerful ally – her grandfather who had died. Sarah was now looking for new allies – her younger sister was one potential candidate as Sarah was able to confide in her on a few occasions. An important discovery with respect to lying was that Sarah's parents perceived it as a kind of failure. Not all family members regarded it in the same way. For example, Sarah's grandfather never used to consider lying as anything more than usual teenage behaviour. It was another discovery that Sarah almost never used to lie to him.

As the session progressed, both Sarah and her mother identified several instances when Sarah was being truthful even under significant threat of punishment.

Sarah also confided that she frequently had thoughts about harming herself by taking tablets but was in control of these thoughts most of the time. Despite the ideas of self-harm trying hard to control her, she managed to stay in charge by telling herself she can do it, by listening to her favourite music and watching comedy movies. She also found painting to be a particularly strong ally in her fight with thoughts of self-harm. Self-harm thoughts and lying were seen as strong allies.

The session ended with Sarah agreeing to notice the times when she was in charge of lying and her mother noticing when Sarah was creative and open.

Understanding Letter

Dear Sarah

I wanted to write you this letter for several reasons. First, I'd like to thank you and your parents for helping me understand your situation better and for working hard to develop an understanding of the challenges your family faces. I enclose the diagram with this letter – did I get the 'exits' from the diagram right? We only managed to discuss the exits for self-harming thoughts: listening to music, watching comedy movies and saying to yourself 'I can do it'. I was wondering if I should have picked up more on another possible exit – your communication skills. Your father mentioned how you help when things get tough between your parents and your sisters. I probably should have asked you more about how you use these skills when things get difficult between your parents and you or even when you face conflicts outside of the family.

I thought your description of lying and self-harm thoughts as your biggest enemies was spot on. You have mentioned how you get into trouble when lying is in charge and how it does not always win. You have sadly lost your grandfather, one of your key allies in the fight against lying. It felt like it was a big loss and your fight got a little more difficult. Self-harm thoughts celebrated a temporary victory when you took the overdose, but you did not give up. You even emerged stronger as your sister could become your close ally and now it sounded like your parents also wanted to be on your side.

Sarah, as you know I have made an appointment to see you next week. I would be very interested to learn more about the times when you are winning against lying and self-harming thoughts. If you notice these times, we could then do some work to discover more about what works best for you and how you can grow even stronger in the future.

With best regards,

Toby Zundel

Summary

A systemic–narrative approach could be adapted to create exits from TA diagrams. TA diagrams could be thought of as descriptions of problem-saturated narratives. Enhancing non-dominant narratives, externalising target behaviours and identifying unique outcomes could all provide opportunities to break the vicious cycles identified.

References

1. Tomm K. Interventive interviewing: Part I. Strategizing as a fourth guideline for the therapist. *Family Process* 1987;26(1):3–13.
2. Selvini M, Boscolo L, Cecchin G, *et al.* Hypothesizing – circularity – neutrality: three guidelines for the conductor of the session. *Family Process* 1980;19(1):3–12.
3. White M, Epston D. *Narrative means to therapeutic ends.* W.W. Norton, 1990: p. 56.

CHAPTER 18

USING COGNITIVE–BEHAVIOURAL THERAPY TECHNIQUES

Audrey Ng

Introduction

Originally developed by Aaron Beck,[1] cognitive–behavioural therapy (CBT) is now regarded to be an effective treatment with a good evidence base in many psychiatric disorders. In this chapter the authors focus on those techniques developed in CBT that can be used in the therapeutic assessment (TA) of young people. We will provide an overview of CBT principles before providing an algorithm of the application of CBT techniques in TA.

The basic idea of CBT is that our thoughts, feelings, behaviours and bodily sensations are all interlinked. All of these elements are found in TA diagrams and therefore could be targets for interventions and exits.

We will describe two CBT interventions that could be used to establish exits from Figure 18.1: cognitive restructuring (targeting thoughts) and behavioural scheduling (targeting behaviour). Relaxation techniques are described in Chapter 21 (targeting bodily sensations).

The cognitive model

Before describing the concept of thought challenging we will briefly review the CBT conceptualisation of thoughts in general.

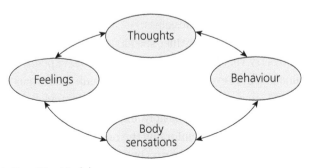

Figure 18.1 Basic Cognitive Model.

Core beliefs are the most general and fundamental ideas held by the young people about themselves, others and the world. Examples of core beliefs may include the following:

- I am unlovable
- I am worthless
- I am unlikable.

These core beliefs may operate at times when a person is depressed, in high anxiety situations or they may be active most of the time. When they are activated, the young person views and interprets the world through the lens of these beliefs. They are global, rigid and overgeneralised. They form a part of the core pain in a TA diagram and give rise to procedures.

Intermediate beliefs consist of rules, attitudes and assumptions that have been derived from the core beliefs.

- I need to constantly please others for them to love me
- I need to work very hard to prove I am worthwhile
- If only I could be cheerful all the time, others will like me.

Elements of intermediate beliefs may form part of procedures in TA diagrams.

Negative automatic thoughts stem from these intrinsic beliefs and are activated by a triggering event.

- My mother hates me (she shouted at me)
- I failed this task (did not have time to finish)
- She doesn't like me (friend brushed passed me at school).

Negative automatic thoughts may form part of procedures in TA diagrams (Figure 18.2).

Example of Lucy

Lucy is a 16-year-old girl who has always felt pressurised by her parents to work hard academically and believed that should she fail at this, she was worthless (core belief) in their eyes. Presently she is struggling at school and this situation has reinforced her core belief of worthlessness.

In order to be perceived as worthwhile, she has an assumption (intermediate belief) that she must always try very hard to please others at the expense of her own needs, but this unsustainable effort eventually leads her to think 'I can't handle this anymore. No one will notice if I am gone. I might as well be dead' (automatic thoughts).

This makes her feel sad and possibly experience a heaviness in her chest (physiological reaction), further reinforcing the negativity that overwhelms her. She may also then be prompted to self-harm (behavioural reaction) to relieve herself from these emotions or even as a sort of punishment for her 'worthless self'.

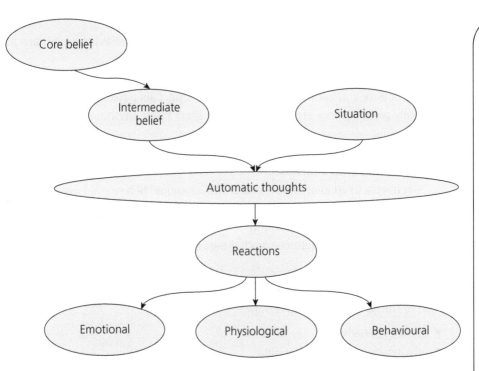

Figure 18.2 The cognitive model.

Identifying cognitive distortions

Distortions of thinking are important to be aware of as they help us to understand how the young person views their internal world. We can view them as 'thinking errors' that prevent the individual from accurately perceiving themselves or the world. Although mainly theoretical constructs, cognitive distortions may inform the process of identifying thoughts as targets.

The main ones are:

- Black and white thinking (dichotomous thinking)
  The tendency to view things in a very all-or-nothing way. It is either a 'complete success' or a 'total failure' with nothing in between.
- Jumping to conclusions (arbitrary inferences)
  Thinking something without any evidence to back it up – e.g. I know he doesn't like me because he did not smile at me when he passed me.
- Catastrophising (fortune telling)
  Predicting the future negatively without considering any other more likely outcomes – I'll be so upset, I won't be able to function at all.
- Overgeneralising
  Allowing an isolated incident to become representative in all other situations – e.g. I did not do well at that exam, I am useless at everything.

- Blaming oneself (personalisation)
  Attributing external events to oneself even though there is little evidence for this – e.g. 'It's my fault that my mother is an alcoholic'.
- Mind reading
  You believe you know what others are thinking, failing to consider other more likely possibilities – He's thinking that I don't know anything at all.
- Labelling
  You put a fixed label on yourself and others – I am stupid. She's useless.
- Should and must statements
  You have a fixed idea of how you or others should behave and overstate how bad it is when these expectations are not met.
- Magnification and minimisation
  A tendency to highlight the 'bad' things that happen and play down the 'good' things that happen.

In the rest of this chapter we will focus on using specific techniques to develop exits from the diagram. We will describe:

- activity scheduling
- challenging negative thoughts
- challenging core pain.

We will use the example of Malcolm to illustrate the techniques above.

Example of Malcolm

Malcolm is a 16-year-old teenager who presented via a GP referral following an escalation of cutting behaviour, with a very deep recent cut that he said was intended to sever his veins.

The precipitating factors for cutting were usually arguments with his mother. She would frequently pass critical comments about Malcolm not doing anything with his life, having a foul mouth and interfering with things that were none of his business. Malcolm on the other hand, acknowledged he was sometimes rude to his mother but thought she was not capable of looking after the family affairs adequately. The latest cut however was precipitated by his girlfriend dumping him, having accused him of being awful in bed and a 'cutting freak'. This made him feel useless and a failure.

Malcolm's parents separated when he was one year old. There is no contact with his father who suffers from a psychotic illness. Malcolm could not recall the last time the relationship between him and his mother was good. He feels she is a pest who never leaves him alone.

Despite this, Malcolm admitted experiencing significant anxiety following their arguments, that would invariably affect his sleep. He acknowledged that he used self-harming as a way of helping him control the anger and anxiety stirred up in him by these rows.

Recently he refused to attend college as he feared being ridiculed by other students over his self-harm. He was also certain that his ex-girlfriend had been indiscreet about their sex life, though had no evidence to support his notion. Malcolm ended up spending increasing amounts of time alone in his bedroom playing computer games and neglecting his previous interests of playing football and going out with his friends who all said he was a good laugh to be around.

Malcolm's TA diagram would look something like the following (Figure 18.3).

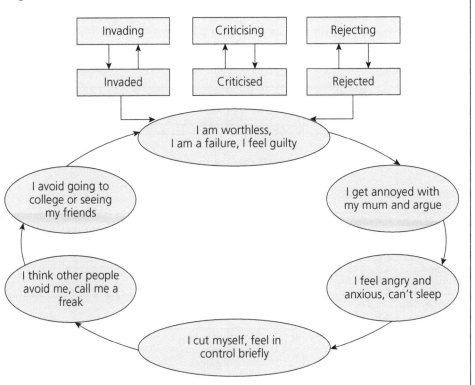

Figure 18.3 Malcolm's diagram.

Activity monitoring and scheduling

In traditional CBT, the activity scheduling charts are filled out and revisited at subsequent sessions. In TA, the aim would be to familiarise the young person with the idea that behaviour can be connected to the way we feel. The young person may find that they are more likely to self-harm when they have been feeling more down in their mood. The types of activities they participate in also have an impact on their self-esteem and confidence which again influences their vulnerability to self-harm.

Key question

Take me through the things you do every day at the moment. Rate the sense of mastery (how skilful you feel doing these activities) and pleasure on a scale from 0 to 10 when you do these activities.

> *Take me through the things you did yesterday. Rate your sense of mastery and pleasure*
> *Rate mastery and pleasure for each activity in your diagram*
> *Rate mastery and pleasure for the activities you are good at*
> *Rate the mastery and pleasure for the activities you used to do but stopped doing now (Tables 18.1 and 18.2).*

Table 18.1 Mastery and pleasure table

Used to do a lot of	Mastery (skill) 0–10	Pleasure 0–10	Do a lot of now	Mastery (skill) 0–10	Pleasure 0–10

0 = no sense of mastery/pleasure.
10 = the strongest sense of mastery/pleasure you have ever experienced.

Table 18.2 Malcolm's example

Used to do a lot of	Mastery (skill) 0–10	Pleasure 0–10	Do a lot of now	Mastery (skill) 0–10	Pleasure 0–10
Playing football	7	9	Arguing with mum	0	0
Socialising	8	9	Smoking cannabis	2	6
Joking	9	9	Playing computer games	6	8

Key question

Thank you for exploring these activities with me. Could you tell me how you would rate your mood when doing these activities?

> *How did your mood change over the last day/week?*
> *Did it relate to the activities you did? How?*
> *Is there a pattern to your mood?*
> *What activities made you feel better? Are these activities going to benefit you in the long term?*
> *What activities made you feel bad? Why? Are these activities going to benefit you in the long term?*

> *What activities can you plan to do so that you feel better more often?*
> *What have you learnt from this exercise?*
> *I/one of my colleagues will see you in the next few days. What activity that gives you a good sense of mastery and pleasure do you think you are most likely to try and do?*
> *How/what/who with/where/when will you do it?*

If you drew the relationship between activity and mood, it might look something like the following (Figure 18.4).

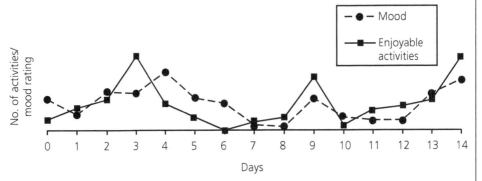

Figure 18.4 Relationship between activity and mood.

Challenging negative thoughts

Key question

What is the evidence to support this thought?
What is the evidence against it?

> *What thought is pushing you around in this situation?*
> *How much do you believe this thought?*
> *How does this thought make you feel?*
> *What is likely to happen if you think that way?*
> *What will I do differently if I stop thinking this way?*
> *What are other ways of seeing this situation? What is the evidence?*
> *What are the other possible explanations? What is the evidence?*
> *What are other ways of seeing yourself?*
> *How would another person see this situation?*
> *What thoughts might they have?*
> *How might these thoughts make them feel?*
> *What would you say to your best friend if he was in the same situation?*

Table 18.3 might help in thought challenging.

Table 18.3 Thought challenging

Circumstances	Describe what was happening for you. Who? Where? What?
Emotions	List the emotions you felt and rate how strongly you felt each of them (0–100%)
Automatic thoughts	List all the thoughts going through your mind at the time. Rate how strongly each one felt for you (0–100%)
Evidence for	Look for factual evidence supporting your belief in these thoughts. (May be easier to pick one or two to concentrate on)
Evidence against	Look for factual evidence that does not support your belief in these thoughts
Other possibilities	Weigh up the evidence and see if there could possibly be a different way of viewing the situation – other points of view. Rate how much you believe them (0–100%)
Re-rate original emotions	Now go back to the original emotions you felt and re-rate them with a balanced view in mind, and see if you still feel as strongly about them

Challenging unhelpful thoughts can be done at any level (core beliefs, intermediate beliefs or negative automatic thoughts), although negative automatic thoughts are usually the most accessible. See Table 18.4 for Malcolm's example.

Table 18.4 Malcolm's example in thought challenging

Circumstances	I was having an argument with my girlfriend. She wanted me to stop cutting. We shouted at each other a lot
Emotions	Anger (99). Ashamed (80)
Automatic thoughts	She thinks I am a freak (80). She doesn't care about me (90). Everyone hates me (80)
Evidence for	She's always nagging me and is on my mother's side. She doesn't appreciate how hard it is for me. She shouted at me and said nasty things
Evidence against	We have been going out for a long time. We were having a nice time before the argument – she bought me cinema tickets. She has told me in the past she loves me
Other possibilities	She may have wanted me to get help (60). She shouted those things because she was angry (70)
Re-rate original emotions	Anger (50). Ashamed (50)

This demonstrated to Malcolm that there can be a more balanced view of bad situations and that taking a moment to think about things made him feel less angry and ashamed.

Challenging core pain: developing a responsibility pie

This technique is useful if there are some strong negative feelings as part of the core pain, particularly if the young person experiences self blame, guilt and undue responsibility for negative outcomes.

Key question

What other things could be responsible for the problem?

> *Who else could be responsible? Anyone else?*
> *Why?*
> *Let's make a pie chart – could you say how much of the responsibility is with the first person/thing you have identified? Second? etc*
> *How much of the responsibility is still with you?*

Example of Malcolm (continued)

Therapist: You mentioned you feel guilty about the arguments with your ex-girlfriend.

Malcolm: Yeah, that's why she dumped me.

Therapist: What were they about?

Malcolm: Erm…, she always wanted to go out and have fun, but I really couldn't do it with my GCSEs coming soon.

Therapist: It sounds like GCSEs are responsible for the arguments a bit, is that right?

Malcolm: Well, I guess so.

Therapist: How much in this pie chart of responsibility do you think the GCSE's share is?

Malcolm: This much (pointing to the chart).

Therapist: What other things were responsible?

Malcolm: Well my mum didn't help and of course my girlfriend wasn't all that reasonable.

In the end, Malcolm's share of responsibility moved from 100 per cent to about 15 per cent (Figure 18.5). Be aware that this process is not about externalising blame but about achieving a realistic appreciation of the situation.

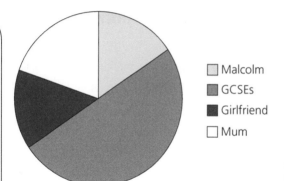

Figure 18.5 Malcolm's share of responsibility.

Challenging core pain: developing an alternative view of the inner self

One technique with which to challenge core pain is to develop a scale of the core pain ideas.

Key question

On a scale from 0 to 10 where 0 is the most (identified core pain) and 10 is the complete opposite, tell me, where do you see yourself? For example, on a scale from 0 to 10 where 0 is being the most worthless and 10 being the most worthwhile, where do you see yourself?

> *Can you think of the most (core pain e.g. unlikable) person in the world as being 0? Can you think of the most (opposite of core pain e.g. likable) person in the world as being 10? Where do you see yourself?*
> *Why not 0?*
> *What evidence do you have? What did it take to achieve it?*
> *Where would your best friend see you on the scale?*
> *Where would (important other) see you on the scale?*
> *Why not 0?*
> *What evidence would they have? What did it take to achieve it?*

Assessment Manual

Example of Malcolm (continued)

Therapist:	On a scale from 0 to 10 where 0 is being the most worthless and 10 being the most worthwhile, where do you see yourself?
Malcolm:	About three.
Therapist:	Why not 0?
Malcolm:	Erm... dunno, I guess I can be quite helpful.
Therapist:	What evidence is there to support this?
Malcolm:	Well, I've managed to fix a washing machine the other day.
Therapist:	Really? What did it take to do it?
Malcolm:	It wasn't easy. It took me a while to figure it out.
Therapist:	So what does it say about you?
Malcolm:	I guess I am quite persistent.
Therapist:	If I were to ask your mother to tell me, what did it take to fix the washing machine, what might she say?
Malcolm:	Don't know, you'd better ask her. She can't fix nothing anyway. She thinks I'm clever because I fixed it.
Therapist:	So it seems there is evidence that you are a persistent and clever person.

Key question

Thank you for exploring these issues with me. Can we go back to the diagram now? Let's imagine that you are more aware of being (name the qualities identified in the challenging core pain exercise e.g. persistence). How might a person with these qualities respond when they feel (lower reciprocal role e.g. criticised)?

> *What might they do next?*
> *What might they do instead of (identified stage in the procedural cycle, e.g. smoking cannabis)?*
> *How might this new way of responding make them feel?*
> *What thoughts might that person have?*
> *How might other people respond when this happens?*

Bearing in mind that not all of the techniques described will be feasible in one session, Malcolm's potential procedures and exits may look something like the following (Figure 18.6).

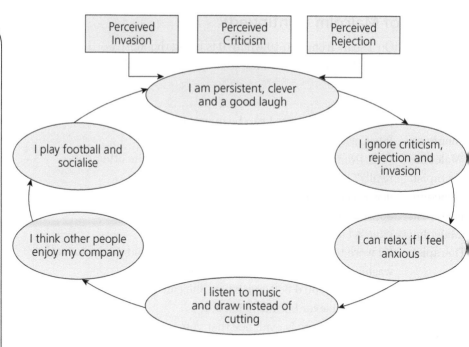

Figure 18.6 Malcolm's example.

Towards the end of the session the therapist undertook a breathing exercise that Malcolm wanted to try and use before going to sleep (see Chapter 21).

Understanding Letter

Hi Malcolm

Following our meeting, I reviewed my notes and discovered how much I have learned about you within that short period of time. Thank you very much for sharing your personal story with me. I am enclosing the two diagrams that we put together. If you have time you might like to have a look at them again and let me know if they still make sense next time we meet. It seemed to me that you have put quite a lot of effort into trying to discover the best ways of breaking the negative cycle of the first diagram. I was very keen to learn more about some of your strengths, like being persistent and smart. You thought that dealing with negative events like criticism might be easier if you hold these strengths in mind. You also thought that doing some of the activities you are good at (like playing football, socialising and sharing jokes) is likely to lift your mood and you thought of doing more of these things in the future. The first thing that came to your mind was for you to play football next Saturday in Wells Park. I hope it isn't raining – would you still play if it did?

Just wanted to let you know about the breathing exercise we did at the end of our meeting. I forgot to tell you that as with any other activity, breathing exercises take time to master. If you like we could also practise this next time we meet.

See you next Tuesday.

With best regards,

Audrey

In summary, using CBT-based approaches offers an opportunity to create exits at several points in the young person's diagram. They are particularly powerful for introducing the young person to the way in which their thoughts, behaviours, physiological reactions and feelings are influencing one another. Detailed examples of the techniques that target negative thoughts, behaviours and bodily responses have been provided. Perhaps the most important technique is challenging core pain – it may provide a new way of interpreting reciprocal role enactments and provide a map for future therapeutic work.

References

1. Beck AT. Thinking and depression: theory and therapy. *Arch Gen Psych* 1964;10:561–71.

CHAPTER 19

USING INTERPERSONAL PSYCHOTHERAPY TECHNIQUES

Paul Wilkinson

Matthias Schwannauer

Introduction

Interpersonal psychotherapy (IPT) was initially developed in the late 1970s in Canada as an individual structured short-term therapy for depressed individuals. It did not arise out of complex theories of how depression is caused. It was instead developed inductively based on clinical practice and the observed needs of depressed individuals. It is a pragmatic treatment, based on the observation that clinical depression often occurs in an interpersonal context, and so improving the interpersonal context should improve the depression. This chapter will begin by describing the process of IPT and move on to describe how IPT principles can be a helpful part of therapeutic assessment.

Interpersonal psychotherapy

Like cognitive–behavioural therapy (CBT), IPT has as its core a model involving a few boxes and a few arrows. However, it is much simpler than the CBT model described in a previous chapter. While this simplicity may be seen as a weakness by some, it is certainly a strength. Our experience has shown us that many young people, who had previously been confused by the CBT model, understand and can relate to the IPT model (Figure 19.1).

To illustrate, what happens in our interpersonal relationships influences our emotions (deeper feelings) and affect (moment to moment feelings). So an argument

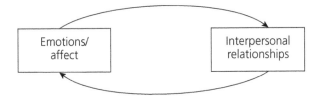

Figure 19.1 Interpersonal psychotherapy model.

with their mother may cause intense feelings of sadness and anger in a young person. In addition, our emotions/affect influence our relationships. So if somebody feels persistently sad, they may stop going out with their friends, and so these friendships may weaken.

Interpersonal psychotherapy works on both components of this cycle. Improving interpersonal relationships should improve emotions and affect. As emotions become more positive, interpersonal relationships should improve. For this to all work, it is crucial that patients are able to recognise these links and to understand what their emotions are, for example to tell the difference between anxiety and anger. Clearly not every problem can be fully dealt with under this formulation, but as depression is multifactorial, removing enough of the causes is likely to drag the patient out of the vicious cycle of depression.

Interpersonal psychotherapy tends to last 12 sessions for adolescents. It has three phases. In the initial, assessment stage, a very important and unique component is the 'Interpersonal Inventory', where the therapist gathers details on all of the important people in the patient's life and the history and details of these relationships. As well as the practicalities of the relationships (e.g. where/how often do you see each other, what do you do together?), the therapist needs to find out about the quality of these relationships: what are the satisfactory and unsatisfactory aspects? What does each member expect from the relationship? Are these expectations reciprocal? If not, there will be, or probably soon will be, problems – here we have IPT's favourite jargon phrase: non-reciprocal role expectations. Does the patient want the relationship to change, and if so, how?

At the end of the assessment phase, the therapist and patient together agree a major focus of the problems, which will be worked on in greater detail in the middle phase. The founders of IPT worked out that interpersonal problems can probably be split into four areas (Box 19.1).

In the middle phase, multiple techniques are used to help the patient recover. At this point it is important to remember that IPT is a pragmatic treatment and that it is understood that changes in the person's depression are brought about by changes in key relationships. This includes the reduction of negative aspects in key relationships but also the fostering and enhancement of positive aspects. At all points, the therapist helps the patient to make the links between emotions/affect and interpersonal events/relationships. These links can operate at various levels, on a moment to moment exchange between people, e.g. in an argument as well as within long-standing and often established patterns in particular relationships, such as with partners or parents. Some techniques are used across foci, while others are more specific. As it is easy for any therapy to wander off into less relevant areas, the therapist tries to keep discussion relevant to the focus area; after all, they and the patient have already concluded that improving the focus is most likely to lead to recovery. Some of the main techniques are described below.

Box 19.1

The four foci of interpersonal psychotherapy

1. Interpersonal disputes
Frequent disagreements with one or several other important others; e.g. frequent arguments with their mother

2. Role transitions
A difficult change from one interpersonal role to another; e.g. moving from America (where the patient was active and popular) to Britain (where they have no friends, and the weather is lousy)

3. Grief
The death of a significant person (or pet)

4. Interpersonal sensitivities
Either a lack of relationships, or a repeated maladaptive pattern of acting in relationships (that stops relationships from being deep and fulfilling)

Develop emotional literacy

To be able to understand the links between emotions and relationships, and between emotions and affect, patients need to know what their emotions are and how they are triggered. As the patient describes interpersonal situations, the therapist needs to try to elicit what their feelings were, and, if necessary, educate them about what the feelings are and how they can change. The goal of this is that a patient can recognise and label affect at the moment it changes (e.g. as anger comes on during an argument).

Encouragement of affect

This refers to acknowledgement and acceptance of unpleasant affect about painful experiences or issues. It also includes the encouragement for individuals to use their affective responses in situations to understand and communicate difficulties in a particular relationship; to recognise how their feelings influence their communications and responses to others and to let people know how they feel.

Improve communication skills

Poor communication is at the root of much interpersonal unhappiness, and arguments. Techniques include: helping the patient to express their unhappiness with an interpersonal situation and making their expectations clear; developing empathy, so they see the other person's point of view. It is often helpful to get exact details of an argument (not just what was said, but also what affects were experienced when – including the patient's guess at the other person's affect). The patient and therapist can then look at what could have been done better – and how this would have led to more positive affect and interpersonal outcomes. The key in this intervention lies in the detail of the exchange, rather than the person's summary or their report of the outcomes.

Role play

When trying to work on improving an adolescent's communication, it can really help to practise it in the session. So you could go back to the beginning of an argument and then get the patient to try acting in a new (hopefully better) way. If you feel brave, swapping roles can be really powerful – the therapist plays the patient in both the unhelpful style and the more positive communication style.

Problem solving

Practical problem solving pops up in all good therapies, including IPT. Not surprisingly, it has already been covered in this book (Chapter 16).

Forming a balanced view of the past and future

Where grief or role transition are the focus, the patient is likely to be grieving the past, which they may see as all good, and dreading the future, which they may see as all bad. These opinions may be too extreme. Help them to mourn their loss, but also to see the positives and negatives of the lost role/person (it is important to be really sensitive here). Then help them to see both the positives and negatives of the future, and help them to make it more positive, in particular by making positive new interpersonal relationships.

Dissolution

Some relationships are beyond repair. You can try to improve things, but sometimes you need to eventually give up and end the relationship. This can cause some short-term grief, but save long-term pain. If a patient no longer cares about a relationship, it has much less power to hurt them. Finding constructive ways of ending relationships is important and requires thought.

Modelling

Acting is more powerful than telling. If you are trying to encourage a patient to act in a certain way, then make sure you act this way. This particularly applies to the communication of affect and sensitivity to affective change in communications; areas that clients with interpersonal problems often find especially difficult.

Transference

Interpersonal psychotherapy therapists are not afraid of transference and acknowledge that it occurs, albeit at a limited level in view of the shortness of therapy. Using it well can be helpful, but needs to be done carefully and with good supervision, otherwise it may do more harm than good.

After the middle phase, the patient will hopefully feel a lot better. In the termination phase, useful strategies from the middle phase are reviewed and consolidated; ending is discussed openly; and warning signs for (and actions to be taken in case of) relapse are discussed. Young people who communicate a range of interpersonal difficulties and low mood often present with underlying insecurities and underdeveloped interpersonal skills and competencies. Many of these interpersonal difficulties may therefore be long-standing or have their roots in earlier negative experiences. That means that the very skills that we may rely on in establishing the interpersonal inventory and in using the described IPT techniques (such as insight, emotional literacy and sensitivity to how the other person may be feeling or what they may be thinking) cannot be taken for granted. These underlying difficulties however can be very significant and often create an emotional resonance in current relationships and interpersonal situations. The responses of the patient to a particular situation can often be explained by emotions that are associated with and resonate with past experiences. This may explain, for example, how a minor rejection experience with a peer can trigger an extreme reaction, i.e. self harming; this needs to be understood in the context of past experiences of rejection or neglect. A carefully taken interpersonal inventory can help you and the patient to understand these patterns and associations of interpersonal experiences in the past and current difficulties in significant relationships. However within a short-term intervention (and certainly within TA) we would not attempt to resolve such underlying attachment difficulties or interpersonal problems and experiences in the past. Instead, we should focus on the key current relationships and set achievable goals.

Interpersonal psychotherapy and family therapy

Those of you trained in family therapy may think: hang on, a lot of these interpersonal problems occur in families, and we already have a great therapy that deals with intrafamilial problems. You are, of course, correct. But not all families will accept the need for change. And family therapy won't deal with peer problems. In fact, even in families who engage well with family therapy, IPT can be of additional benefit to the index case, to help them to think about their relationships without other family members in the room. We quite often use family therapy alongside IPT, and this combination can work well.

Interpersonal psychotherapy in the therapeutic assessment

Research has demonstrated that 12 sessions of good-quality IPT is more effective than control treatments in treating adolescent depression.[1–3] Clearly, we cannot deliver 12 sessions at a post-self-harm assessment. But we do believe that we can use the techniques of IPT to improve this therapeutic assessment.

Many acts of self-harm follow acute interpersonal events – commonly arguments (especially with parents) and also rejections. They can also occur in the context of chronic interpersonal difficulties, such as bullying, a lack of friends, poor family relationships and grief.[4,5] So enquiring in detail about these interpersonal problems is likely to improve our understanding of the young person's predicament. This will improve the quality of the assessment; but, in addition, by helping the young person to feel more understood, it should improve engagement. Then trying to improve these interpersonal problems is likely to improve the young person's predicament, reducing the risk of future self-harm.

Interpersonal psychotherapy techniques can therefore be used at two levels in the therapeutic assessment (TA). First, we can use techniques from the interpersonal inventory to improve the shared understanding of interpersonal relationships, leading to a more accurate TA diagram. Second, techniques used in the middle phase of IPT can be used to help the young person to break out of the vicious cycle identified in the TA diagram.

We will now describe an algorithm of an IPT-based 'exit' followed by an in-depth case discussion.

Interpersonal psychotherapy – therapeutic assessment algorithm

I. Constructing a closeness cycle

I would like to ask you some questions about the important people in your life and about your relationships with them. First of all, let's make a list of those people: A, B, C and D. [At this point, we can use either a closeness circle or a spider diagram.]

Now I'd like to ask you to place these people on this 'closeness circle'. The star in the middle is you and the closer the relationship with you the closer on the circle the person should be (Figure 19.2).

Now I'd like to ask you to imagine that you are in the middle of this 'spider diagram'. The closer the relationship with you the closer to you the person should be on the diagram (Figure 19.3). We can draw lines between people who have links with each other.

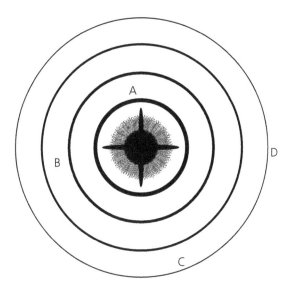

Figure 19.2 Closeness circle.

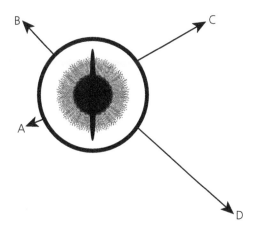

Figure 19.3 Spider diagram.

In order to establish the link of the young person's key relationships to their mood and, specifically, self-harming episodes, it is important to ascertain the quality of these particular relationships. It is important to have a full exploration of the key relationships in terms of impact on mood/self-harming. The following questions are some examples of how to establish the potential impact of these relationships.

II Choosing the target relationship(s)

Which of these relationships is the most important to you?
Which of these relationships has caused you to feel very upset or angry at times?
Which of these relationships have been affected most by self-harm?
Which of these relationships would you most like to change?

III Exploring the target relationship with A

What are the good things about A?
What are the not so good things about A?
What are the good things about your relationship?
What are not so good things about it?
When does the relationship work best?
When does the relationship work worst?
Do you ever talk with A about your feelings?
What things about your relationship would you like to change? Why?
Do you think there are any aspects of the relationship that A would like to change. Why?
What things about your relationship do you think should remain as they are? Why?

IV Exploring interpersonal role disputes

Are there things that you and A do not agree on? What are they?
What happens when you try to talk about them?
How do you feel then? What do you do? What is it that A does that upsets you?
How do you think A feels then? What does s/he do? Is there anything that you do that upsets A?
Do you ever let A know how you feel?
Do you ever acknowledge how A might feel?
What do you think happens when people don't acknowledge their feelings?

/ Setting targets

> *What might improve your relationship with A?*
> *What may be the first little thing you could do to improve the relationship?*
> *What might you do differently during the arguments?*
> *What would happen if you let A know how you feel?*
> *What would happen if you acknowledged how A might feel?*
> *What would happen if you offered a compromise? What might that compromise be?*
> *How might your relationship change if you were doing more nice things together? What might those things be?*
> *How might your relationship change if you offered to do something nice to A for no reason? What might that thing be?*

/I Closing the intervention

We have been talking about your relationship with A for a while and you had some really good ideas about how this relationship might improve. When I see you next time (give time, date and place) we might discuss this relationship some more and you could also tell me if you noticed any changes in that relationship.

Clinical example: Karen

Let us consider the example of Karen, a 15-year-old girl from a white middle-class family. Her father is a lawyer in a top financial institution and her mother is a merchant banker. Both parents have always worked long hours, and have always employed nannies to look after the children. At the most, each nanny would last a year, and Karen would not know why they would leave. Her parents have always been strict. They have always made her work hard at school, and have emphasised the importance of getting good qualifications. Over the last year or two, she has been teased by her friends for not being allowed out so much, and for working so hard at school. She feels that some friends have started to get more distant from her. She has responded to this by trying to push the boundaries at home, working less and going out more. This has led to arguments with her parents. This has led to her feeling increasingly trapped, not able to please either her parents or her friends at the same time. After an argument with her parents for coming back late one night, Karen took an overdose of 16 paracetamol tablets. This was partly because she felt as if she was trapped and had an impulsive wish to die as a way out, and partly to hurt her parents for being so strict.

Now, the readers might like to think of the key elements of Karen's diagram before looking at the authors' version below (Figure 19.4).

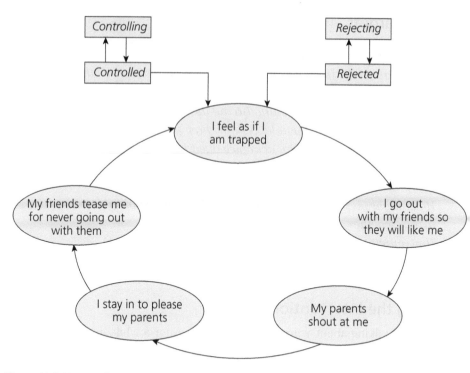

Figure 19.4 Karen's diagram.

Here's one possible version of the diagram. Karen described a predominant feeling – core pain – of feeling as if she were trapped between her parents and friends; and an underlying insecurity that she may not or may be able to give enough as a person to either of them. In terms of reciprocal roles, there are at least two controlled-controlling, with both parents and friends trying to tell her what to do, then Karen eventually snapping by taking an overdose to get them back. Secondly rejecting-rejected, with Karen feeling rejected by her parents who she felt never spent much time with her throughout her life, by her nannies for leaving her, and her friends for turning against her, leading to an attempt to kill herself and so reject the other people in her life (Figure 19.4).

To take this assessment further it is important to gather as much relevant interpersonal information as possible in the short assessment. The relationship that led acutely to the overdose was that with the parents. So try to find out more about this relationship – in fact find out about these relationships, as there are two parents! When do they argue? What makes them argue? How often do they argue? But also ask about the strengths of the relationships; do they have fun together? Are the parents supportive? Remember, we want to know about positive and negative aspects and any exceptions to the usual patterns. Now, let's get deeper; arguments happen because the parents want Karen to stay in and work. Why does Karen think they do this? Is it because they want *what they think* is the best for her? What do they think is best for her? What role do they think Karen should play? But what is the problem with this? What does Karen think is best? What role does Karen think she should have? And here we get to the nub of the problem: Karen thinks her parents see her role as being a hard-working high-achieving daughter, who will get wonderful grades, go to university and get a high-flying job (like them). When we ask them, they confirm this: 'Of course that's what we think, what caring parent wouldn't?' Karen sees her role as being a rounded teenager, who does OK at school, but who is popular and well-liked by her friends.

Karen's friends are 'normal teenagers' (Karen's words). They want to go out and have fun lots, and don't seem so bothered by work. They have also always been a bit bitchy, and have always slagged off girls outside their group. Now Karen isn't always with them, they are starting to see her as 'outside the group', and a target for bitching. Karen thinks they see her role (and all the group's role) as a loyal member of the group who will always hang around with the others. Karen sees her role as different. She actually does love her parents (speaking about the positives of their relationships brought out some lovely descriptions and feelings), and wants to spend time with them (they do have some fun together). She also wants to do well at school (but not at the cost of everything else). And she wants to have fun with her long-term friends. Again, she sees her role as being a rounded teenager, who does OK at school, but who is popular and well-liked by her friends.

What do we have here? Let's get down to some IPT jargon (one of very few bits of jargon in IPT!) We have some non-reciprocal role expectations. Karen has different opinions of what her roles should be than her parents, on one hand, and her friends, on the other. In fact, her parents and friends have diametrically-opposite opinions, and they let Karen know it. And Karen feels as if she is trapped in the middle (Figure 19.5).

Using interpersonal therapy techniques

Hopefully Karen will now understand her problems better, and feel better understood by us. But the next thing she says might be: 'Well, that all makes lots of sense. But I am stuck here trapped in the middle of it, and can't see any way of things getting any better.' So now it's time to use some IPT techniques to get some exits.

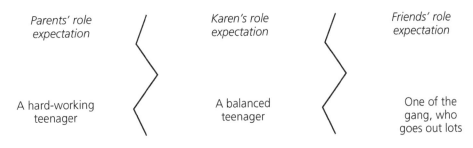

Parents' role expectation

Karen's role expectation

Friends' role expectation

A hard-working teenager

A balanced teenager

One of the gang, who goes out lots

Figure 19.5 Karen's feelings of being trapped.

Let us now update the TA diagram (Figure 19.6).

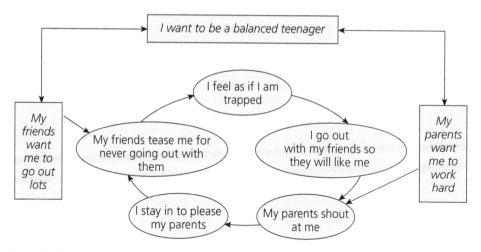

Figure 19.6 Karen's updated diagram.

Please try to think what we could do. Where is change possible in this diagram and how could we facilitate this? How could Karen act differently? Think about what the consequences could be of all these different possible solutions.

Karen clearly feels as if she is trapped in the middle between her parents' and friends' role expectations. Of course, one solution is to break one of these bonds – 'dissolution' in IPT-speak. If she did that, the relationships at the other pole would be in a much more harmonious state. But is that really practical? Can she break off from her parents? Well, that seems a bit extreme, especially as she does love them and values lots of things about their relationship. What about these friends? Easier to break away from than her parents, certainly. But how would they react? The history suggests they'd be even more horrible once she was an absolute outsider. Could Karen cope with that? Maybe, if she has a thick skin. But if they are her only friends, she's be left friendless – ouch! A key determinant of whether this would be a good idea is the rest of her interpersonal network.

So what should Karen do? Well, probably the best person to ask is Karen! IPT (and TA) is a collaborative process. Once you have built up your diagram together, and identified the key problems caused by the non-reciprocal role expectations, ask her what her ideas are on how to exit. It is quite likely she will come up with something like, 'I don't know what to do. I really like my friends and I really like my parents. I don't want to hurt any of them, but I don't want things to stay how they are.'

So dissolution isn't really an option. We are left with the other classic option when there is an interpersonal disputes focus: 'renegotiation'. If Karen doesn't want to lose the relationships but doesn't want things to stay the same, she needs to change something. Which relationship? One of them, both of them? Ask Karen. One may be easier than the other.

Of course, you have the backup of your friendly family therapist in the long run if she wants to change things with her parents. But in the TA, that is your job.... You can certainly engage the parents in looking at this. The parents may not see any problem right now, in which case you and Karen need to think together about what to do about this. She may want to work on the relationship with her friends instead. She may want to do both (here, you are really likely to be running into time troubles, so it may be best to try to focus on one thing).

Several IPT techniques could be helpful here. Firstly, Karen has a big decision to make. What will she do about the relationship in question? She has several options, and you need to think together about what they are, and weigh up the pros and cons. A big issue is the conflicting role expectations. Karen may have never thought about it before meeting us. Her parents/friends probably haven't either. So what about her discussing it with them? The heat of the next argument is probably not the best time. A calm time where there is space to talk is better. After the overdose when people are concerned about her may be a good opportunity to get a sympathetic ear.

But how? Karen may be terrified about the thought of telling people she wants them to act differently. It will really help her if you think about how to do it together. Maybe some role play will help. However it is done, it is important to remember the goal of this conversation: they are in conflict, and this is partly because they have different expectations of Karen. Both sides need to listen to and understand the opposite's expectations (remember: Karen could have been wrong!) IPT is an affect-based therapy and this principle may help at this critical point. For Karen to communicate clearly how she feels in situations may facilitate openness and transparency in the dialogue; it is also something that others usually find difficult to argue with. It is important that the young person is assertive here; that they state how they feel and what they want clearly, but without being aggressive, making the other person annoyed and defensive, and starting another argument. Hopefully both sides will then come up with a solution together. Here is an example of what might happen:

Karen:	Mum, we've been arguing a lot recently and at those times I feel sad and stuck.
Mum:	I know, and I wish we weren't. I really hate having to shout at you.
Karen:	And we both know that I took the overdose after one of our arguments.
Mum:	I know, and I feel so bad about that. I wish so much that we hadn't argued like that, but then that seems to be the only way we talk at the moment.

Karen: It is, and I wish it wasn't. I've been doing some thinking about these arguments with the psychiatrist who saw me after the overdose. We tried to work out why these arguments happen.

Mum: Your dad and I have also been thinking about it. They always seem to happen when you come in late, or don't do what we want you to do.

Karen: Please don't start on me again. I know that's why we argue, it's obvious.

Mum: OK, OK. I guess this will be easier if we both stay calm.

Karen: Yes, it will. We were trying to think about the arguments, and how they are always about the same thing. It seems we have different opinions of what my life should be like.

Mum: I agree with you on that one.

Karen: Well, maybe we should each talk about what we want from my life.

Mum: OK. Well, I think you need to work hard. Your GCSEs are next year and you really need to do well. You don't want to be wasting your time with those friends of yours. They are going to get you into big trouble one day.

[Karen now has a golden opportunity to let another big argument develop. But you'll be amazed how young people with a bit of IPT training can do better than that.]

Karen: I know how you really want me to do well, and that you think my friends aren't helping me. I know it is because you love me and want the best from me. And I really appreciate how much you care.

[To stop a nasty argument developing, it is really important to acknowledge the other side's opinions before saying your own. We would thoroughly recommend a Juliet Capulet approach: in Romeo and Juliet, Juliet's father tells her he has arranged a marriage for her with Paris, when she secretly loves Romeo. Rather than storm off in a sulk, she humbly tells her father that she is, 'Not proud you have, but thankful that you have. Proud can I never be of what I hate, But thankful even for hate that is meant love.'[6] Let the other know you appreciate their efforts and their loving motives on the one hand; but make it very clear you think their decision is wrong.]

Mum   [who is a bit taken aback, and is no longer angry]: But we do care, love. we just want the best for you.

Karen   [who must now grab her opportunity of a receptive audience and deliver the 'not proud']: But I am now getting older and am starting to think about what I want from my life. I do want to work hard and get good exam grades [start with the agreement stuff, to keep mum on side], but I also think that other things are important in my life, and I do want some balance in my life. My friends are important to me, and we have lots of fun together. I think that it is important I let my hair down occasionally, and then I think my work will be better, because I'm all refreshed [think together in advance about any advantages to mum's side about what Karen wants]. I feel like sometimes I can't get things right.

Mum [sweetened a bit by the last two sentences]: I can see what you mean. Maybe we haven't been thinking too much about what you want. Maybe we have been too strict. I suppose you could go out a bit more. You are doing very well at school, after all, and a few more hours out probably won't hurt. Shall we see how it goes? But let's review it at the end of term. If your report shows your grades have slipped, we'll know why, and we'll have to look again at your social life [you didn't really expect this mother to not assert her control at the end, did you?].

So we could well have found an exit. It may work; it may not. You may think this all sounds unrealistic — teenagers don't speak like that. Well, they don't speak like that because they have never learnt how to. Actually, lots of adults don't speak like that. But with some training, they can be taught to — we know, because we have seen it. When your previously socially inept and passive patient comes and tells you that his friends now comment on how amazing and mature he is at sorting out everyone else's interpersonal crises, you'll believe in the power of IPT and have faith in the interpersonal ability of young people.

The dialogue above is the ideal outcome of a therapeutic intervention. What might be the first step Karen could do to achieve this interpersonal competence? Again a good person to ask is Karen. Before your next appointment, could she try one or to new ways of negotiation? Could she acknowledge her feelings as well as the feelings of her parents? Is there a possible point of compromise?

This situation will certainly need follow-up, and your family therapist may come in helpful (possibly more helpful than an individual therapist). But you will have sent Karen out with some hope that life can change. And some hope that child and adolescent mental health services can be helpful, and are worth coming back to see.

In summary, interpersonal therapy works by examining the links between emotions and interpersonal relationships, and by trying to improve each of these. IPT techniques can be used in the therapeutic relationship in two main ways. First, a more accurate TA picture can be built up if a lot of detail is gleaned about key interpersonal relationships. Second, IPT therapeutic techniques can be used to improve a difficult interpersonal situation and to help patients to exit their TA cycle.

References

1. Mufson L, Dorta KP, Wickramaratne P, *et al*. A randomized effectiveness trial of interpersonal psychotherapy for depressed adolescents. *Arch Gen Psychiatry* 2004;61(6):577–84.
2. Mufson L, Weissman MM, Moreau D, Garfinkel R. Efficacy of interpersonal psychotherapy for depressed adolescents. *Arch Gen Psychiatry* 1999;56(6):573–9.
3. Rossello J, Bernal G. The efficacy of cognitive-behavioral and interpersonal treatments for depression in Puerto Rican adolescents. *J Consult Clin Psychol* 1999;67(5):734–45.
4. Hawton K, Fagg J. Deliberate self-poisoning and self-injury in adolescents. A study of characteristics and trends in Oxford, 1976–89. *Br J Psychiatry* 1992;161:816–23.
5. Hawton K, Fagg J, Simkin S. Deliberate self-poisoning and self-injury in children and adolescents under 16 years of age in Oxford, 1976–1993. *Br J Psychiatry* 1996;169(2):202–8.
6. Shakespeare W. The tragedy of Romeo and Juliet, Act III, Scene V. 1595.

CHAPTER 20

MENTALISATION-BASED INTERVENTIONS

Tobias Zundel

Introduction

Mentalisation has been defined as implicitly and explicitly interpreting the actions of oneself and others as meaningful on the basis of intentional mental states. In other words, having the awareness that all people have their own feelings and thoughts (mental states) that determine their actions while, by their very nature, mental states are opaque and can't be 'read' directly.

In its most basic sense this definition of mentalisation describes something that occurs to varying degrees in all human social interactions. One of the aims of therapeutic assessment (TA) in general is that it should be a mentalising intervention. That is to say, clinicians are encouraged to consider mentalisation as being an important underlying component of all meaningful psychotherapeutic work. Hence, they should aspire to maintain an ongoing awareness as to their own degree of mentalising, as well as that of the patient, during their clinical interactions. This has been described as the mentalising stance. Another way of putting it is the ability on the therapist's part to question continually what internal mental states both within their patient and within themselves can explain what is happening now.

Mentalisation-based therapy (MBT) for borderline personality disorder and the description of mentalisation given above were developed by Professor Anthony Bateman and Professor Peter Fonagy as an approach to understanding and working with adults suffering from severe borderline personality disorder. A number of further therapeutic approaches to clinical work have been devised on the conceptual framework of mentalisation. These include short-term mentalisation and relational therapy (SMART), which is described as an integrative family therapy for working with children and adolescents.

The evidence base for the effectiveness of Bateman and Fonagy's MBT for partially hospitalised adults with borderline personality disorder makes it arguably the best treatment approach for these highly complex and difficult-to-manage individuals. An

8-year follow-up study reported clinical and statistical superiority to treatment as usual on suicidality (23 per cent vs 74 per cent) and service use (2 years vs 3.5 years) as well as other favourable outcomes in relation to educational status and global functioning.[1] The studies have also indicated a reduction in self-harming behaviour.

Based on the advancement of attachment theory in developmental psychology, mentalisation is now understood as being a developmental achievement through childhood. Depending, in part, on the manner in which early attachment relationships facilitate this, the process advances with varying degrees of robustness. As adults we are all capable of slipping into non-mentalising states of mind under certain conditions and impaired mentalisation is conceptualised as being the core pathology in borderline personality disorder.

Research that includes neuro-imaging studies suggests that individuals can develop an overactive attachment mechanism (defined neuroanatomically). In the context of an attachment relationship this can then, usually in combination with stress and other states of arousal, result in mentalisation being inhibited. The basis has then been established for spontaneous, aggressive and destructive actions driven by an overwhelming affect storm. Such non-mentalising states of mind are linked to both urges and acts of suicide or self-harm. What is often remarkable about this process is that at other times, or in non-attachment relationships, these individuals can function very well.

Three basic non-mentalising states of mind have been outlined: the mode of psychic equivalence, the teleological stance and the pretend mode. When mentalisation is impaired there is a tendency to 'regress' into one or more of these states.

Mentalisation-based therapy involves continuously trying to identify when a patient is not mentalising in any of these ways, or is giving a historical account of events in which they were clearly not in a mentalising state of mind (the account involves a loss of the mentalising thread). When this occurs, one key component of the therapy is based on a direct intervention at this point. While maintaining a genuinely curious, supportive and empathic position the therapist tries to 'stop and stand', challenging the patient in an attempt to keep the therapist 'on board' and regain mentalisation.

This most basic of strategies can, in common with the more advanced and complex components of the therapy, help the patient practise finding their way back to mentalising, which over time appears to be an effective way of improving interpersonal functioning and self destructive crises.

The three non-mentalising states of mind are described below. Some clinical examples follow later and these can make it easier to understand and recognise what is meant. They all relate to specific early stages in childhood development.

Psychic equivalence

This is mind–world isomorphism. What is experienced as being real in the mind is real in the outside world, regardless of what objective evidence there is to support this. The internal has the power of the external and there is an intolerance of alternative perspectives.

The teleological stance

A physical act is required as proof that something is real. It is not possible to accept anything other than a modification in the realm of the physical as a true index of the intentions of the other. There is a focus on understanding actions in terms of their physical as opposed to their mental constraints.

The pretend mode

Ideas form no bridge between inner and outer reality. The mental world is decoupled from external reality. There is a dissociation of thought with possible pseudo-mentalising.

In MBT the fundamental position the clinician takes is:

- not knowing
- inquisitive
- supportive
- empathic.

A number of increasingly advanced interventions are built up from this basis:

- clarification, challenge and elaboration (including 'stop and stand')
- basic mentalising (including 'stop, look, listen' and 'stop, re-wind, explore')
- interpretative mentalising
- mentalising the transference
- non-mentalising interpretations (to be used with care).

In TA there is no intention to take the therapy to the more advanced levels as it lies both outside of the scope of what is expected within a 15- to 20-minute intervention and cannot be covered in a manual of this size.

Mentalising interventions within therapeutic assessment

The relevance of MBT to TA can be seen on many levels. Most generally the degree of mentalising demonstrated by any young person throughout the assessment process is likely to impact significantly on their ability to establish a rapport and give a coherent history. It could also be a useful indicator of the ongoing level of distress and agitation experienced by the young person during the assessment. In view of this any reliable strategies available to the clinician that facilitate the improvement or regaining of mentalisation could be of benefit.

There is no doubt that during acute assessments following self-harm, especially i
it occurred in the very recent past, young people can be extremely distressed and
emotionally overwhelmed, often experiencing ongoing suicidal ideation or intent. This
can frequently be experienced as a crisis in itself that challenges the assessing clinician
to their limits. It requires them to draw on their deepest resources to contain and
manage the situation. It is in precisely these circumstances, when the patient is also
not mentalising, that certain MBT strategies could be helpful. This will be outlined in
more detail later.

Despite the two points above, the main emphasis in this chapter is the use of a
basic mentalisation intervention as an exit from the TA diagram.

After taking the history and attempting to construct the TA diagram, the degree
to which the young person is mentalising may already be clear. If their history is hard
to follow and appears to contain repeated examples of errors and unjustified
assumptions about the feelings, thoughts and actions of others then it is likely that
mentalising is impaired. As the therapist it is often possible to notice if the patient is
aware that you are trying to follow their story and if you are 'with them' or not. This
can also be a good measure of the actual degree of mentalising that is taking place
there and then.

Step 1: identify if mentalisation is impaired

Key indication: a non-mentalised procedural loop

If the procedural loop that is created together with the young person appears to follow
a non-mentalising logic, i.e. it includes assumptions or 'errors' in understanding
themselves or others, this could be an indicator that a mentalising intervention is
appropriate. A further guide might be if the point on the diagram that is chosen by the
young person specifically relates to such a 'non-mentalising leap' in the flow of events
or narrative.

Certain types of questions help to clarify the quality of a patient's mentalising.
Possible questions are listed below.

Why did your parents behave as they did during your childhood?
*Do you think you, or your friends play a bigger role in shaping
the kind of friendships you have?*
*Do you think your childhood experiences have an influence on
who you are today?*
Did you ever feel rejected as a child?
*With respect to losses, abuse or other trauma, how did you feel at
the time and how have your feelings changed over time?*

Possible examples of how non-mentalising can present:

- excessive details with no mention of motivations, feelings or thoughts;
- emphasis on external social factors like parents, friends or the school;
- emphasis on physical or structural labels like: tired, lazy clever, self-destructive, depressed;
- statements of certainty about thoughts or feelings of others;
- emphasis on fault finding or blaming;
- denial of involvement in problems;
- emphasis on rules, responsibilities, 'shoulds' and 'should nots'.

In general mentalising interventions should be:

- simple
- focused more on the patients' mind and not their behaviour
- affect-focused
- related to current events or activity (if past events are being discussed the focus should be on how the young person thinks and feels about them now in order to encourage current mentalising).

Example of Michael

Michael is a 15-year-old who lives with his mother and stepfather. His parents split up when he was 3 and his mother has been together with his stepfather for 11 years. His stepfather is from Australia and works as an accountant. He works long hours and is very preoccupied with Michael's education and academic progress. He says that term time is work time and feels strongly that Michael should not engage in social activities in the evenings or even weekends, as he has to work towards his exams. Michael feels this is unrealistic and his stepfather is overly intrusive and controlling in relation to his school work. Michael has excellent grades at school but feels like his stepfather thinks he's stupid and isn't doing well enough. Michael's mother suffers from low moods.

Michael's mother and his step father have not been getting on over the last year. Financial problems are the main cause of their arguments. Michael's stepfather has started going to the office at weekends and also goes to football every Saturday. He didn't used to be such a keen fan in the past and the two of them used to go swimming together at weekends.

Michael has two close friends (Dan and James) he's known for years and he dislikes large groups. He was always described as a difficult, emotional child. He started to cut his arms in the past 3 months and presented to the emergency department (ED) after he cut deeper than he had before, requiring stitches. This was after an argument with his stepfather (Figure 20.1).

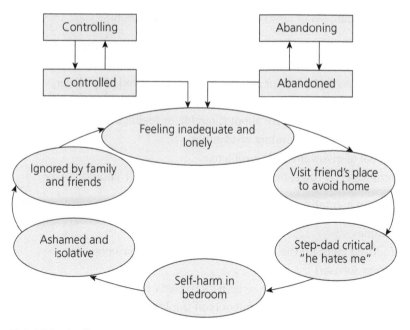

Figure 20.1 Michael's diagram.

Step 2: identify which non-mentalising state of mind is being used

Example of psychic equivalence

Michael tells you:

> *I stayed late at my friends house and then my step-dad grounded me for two weeks. I know he only did that because he hates me and thinks I'm stupid and will never amount to anything.*

Such an occurrence could be described in the language of CBT, see Chapter 18, as a negative automatic thought. These are often very good examples of failures in mentalisation. The indication for the clinician that a mentalisation-based intervention might be the most helpful at addressing such a 'thinking error' is probably going to be related to the overall sense of whether the young person is more psychologically minded or whether they are functioning in a more 'borderline' manner. The research evidence suggests that an MBT approach can be effective at providing a therapeutic experience that facilitates insight and mentalisation in patients who have borderline personality disorder.

Mentalisation-based therapy advocates that the therapist generally tries to step in at the moment when it becomes obvious that the mentalising thread is lost. It is argued that in patients with borderline personality disorder, allowing the patient to just continue when they have essentially 'lost you' is usually counterproductive and can even contribute to potentially harmful therapeutic phenomena.

This example also applies if Michael chooses the stage in the diagram where is stepfather is critical and Michael feels that he hates him as the point at which he wants to intervene or make a change from the usual pattern that leads to him self-harming.

A basic technique implemented at this point is 'Stop and Stand'.

Key question/intervention

'(Michael), I am so sorry to interrupt you there, but I'm afraid you are going to have to help me. I really want to understand what you are explaining about what happened, but I seem to have got a bit confused. Can you take me through it again step by step? (In the example of Michael you might then say) You said that your dad caught you coming in late and obviously wasn't happy, so he grounded you. I could follow that bit, but then you said he did that because .... I just don't quite see how you know that?'

It may be necessary to stick to this point with some persistence until it is addressed in a mentalising way:

> *Bear with me. I think we need to continue trying to understand what was going on.*

It is a challenge to do this and stay empathic. Sometimes it goes wrong and results in serious agitation. The clinician then needs to return to the basic supportive stance while making a mental note of what happened.

It is important that the therapist tries not to undermine mentalising by taking on the role of an 'all-knowing' expert. An extreme example of this might be modelling non-mentalising by stating with certainty what the patient is feeling or thinking.

If any form of therapy offers a causal explanation for an underlying mental state, such a ready-made answer could provide an obstacle to genuine mentalisation. The patient is left with only two options, denial or uncritical acceptance.

Michael goes on to say:

> *It's just so obvious that he hates me. I know it because he now goes to football every weekend just to avoid me.*

This is an example of psychic equivalence as Michael is convinced that his step-dad hates him because of his going to football. Any suggestion that there might be a different reason for his step-dad's actions, for example wanting to get away from Michael's mum, can't be considered by Michael.

Some basic mentalising interventions are explained below.

Stop, listen, look

When mentalisation is impaired during an interaction:

- stop and investigate
- let the interaction unfold slowly while you control it
- highlight who feels what
- identify how each aspect is understood from multiple perspectives
- identify how messages feel and are understood, what reactions occur.

> *What do you think it feels like for (mum/dad) at the weekend?*
> *Can you think of some other ways you could help your dad understand what you feel like?*
> *What do you think (mum/friend Dan) feels is going on when your dad goes to football?*
> *How does your mum react to dad leaving?*

Stop, re-wind, explore

> *Tell me when you first started to feel like you might harm yourself?*
> *When was the last point at which you felt fine? What happened after that? (This could uncover the trigger for self-harm)*
> *Who was around at the time or who were you thinking about?*
> *Hold on, before we move off lets just re-wind and see if we can understand something in all this.*

Example of the teleological stance

In fact Michael goes as far as saying. The only way that his dad could prove to him that he cares is if he stays at home every weekend for a whole month and they start going swimming again. A physical action is required to demonstrate that something is true, or real. Even if Michael's stepfather tells him 50 times that he loves Michael dearly and is the most important thing in the world to him, it means nothing to Michael unless his exact demands for a physical proof are met.

When confronted by the teleological stance, which can also be directed at the clinician, 'To show me that you care about me you have to hold my hand now', it is best to try to avoid the conversation becoming fixed and entrenched around the demand that is being made. Making a definitive comment, either yes or no, in relation to the demanded action tends to be problematic. Often the demand is inappropriate 'I need you to hug me' or 'you can't leave me until the morning' and so saying yes is not an option. Immediately saying no is likely to be experienced as an overwhelming rejection, with potentially serious consequences on any further cooperation.

Ideally the clinician has a sense of the desperation that is underlying the teleological demand and on this basis it is possible to talk around the issue, exploring its complexity without addressing it head on. If this is done in a supportive and empathic manner it is remarkable how quickly the specific demand can become irrelevant or forgotten as the patient regains mentalisation and feels generally more contained and reassured. A danger here is to be drawn into the teleological view and in this way somehow accept a simple solution to what is a complicated issue.

An alternative possibility is to just name or suggest what feelings may be underlying the demand and leaving it at that.

Example of the pretend mode

Michael goes on to tell you that his parents are fighting nearly every day now and that he's really worried about them, especially his mother. He says that he thinks they are going to just keep doing this and he can't see how anything's going to change. He gives examples of really nasty things they say to each other and how they upset each other terribly. He says that last week his mum refused to come out of her room for 2 days and his step-dad slept on the sofa in the lounge. He says he has never seen his step-dad so angry before and he even smashed the TV. Finally, he says he thinks that at this rate they will probably kill each other one of these days.

While listening to this you begin to notice something remarkable about Michael. You realise that he is not demonstrating any congruent affective states or emotions that relate to the things he is saying. He states he is worried about his mother, but he doesn't appear worried. He doesn't seem distressed or upset talking about his step-dad having smashed the TV, or even when telling you he thinks one of his parents could actually kill the other. This is an example of the pretend mode.

Key question: stop, listen, look

That sounds really awful. I think I would be terrified to see an argument like that. How would you feel if something horrific happened to your mum because your step-dad lost control?

What could you/they do to try to ensure that arguments don't get so angry in future?

The focus here is not so much to arrive at an actual solution or answer to the questions raised, but more to just re-establish mentalising on behalf of the patient by means of you using your own curious and empathic thoughts and feelings to gently share and engage with the content of what is being expressed.

Other ways in which the clinician can experience a patient in the pretend mode is when the clinician feels redundant or meaningless. The patient is not really interested or able to make use of the clinician as they apparently rage or complain about their situation extensively in an unmentalising fashion; once again they have 'lost you' and probably have not noticed or perhaps don't care.

Pseudomentalising

A form of this is when patients talk at length about complicated plans and solutions they will implement to solve all of their problems, but you can sense that somehow there is no reality to the planning and it appears like they have said it all before. This kind of pseudomentalising can be very convincing in patients who are intelligent and high functioning. However, it is felt to be generally unhelpful for clinicians to facilitate this kind of interaction over an extended period.

One of the risks is that in the pretend mode patients can talk, almost endlessly, in such a way that valuable time passes and no real therapy is possible as the patient is disconnected from what they are saying, or not mentalising. This is why a mentalising intervention can be very helpful to bring the patient out of the pretend mode again.

Challenging the pretend mode, and especially pseudomentalising in the pretend mode, needs to be done with great care as it can expose an internal void that is potentially intolerable for the patient.

Example of an apparently impossible situation (switch from pretend mode into psychic equivalence)

When a distressed young person places the clinician in an apparently impossible position because of a catastrophic failure of mentalisation during an acute assessment this can be particularly challenging.

Michael has just been recounting that he's started to think even his two friends don't really care about him. It was Dan's birthday at the weekend and they went to the cinema but didn't invite Michael along. Then when he heard them talking about the film yesterday they quickly changed the subject. Michael appeared quite detached while telling this story.

At this point the assessment takes a turn for the worse after the clinician quickly checks the time on their watch, having remembered that Michael's mum was coming in at 11 o'clock.

Michael says:

> *Don't worry I'm not going to take up much more of your time. You obviously have something more important to do somewhere else. I can see you've been getting bored of listening to me. In fact, it's clear now that you don't give a toss about me. You're just like all the rest of them. You're meant to help, but you hate me just like*

everyone else. There's obviously nobody that can help and I've been wasting your time. I might as well just go and kill myself now and it'll be your fault. This is your last chance. How are you going to help me? What are you going to do? If you don't make me feel better that's it.

This kind of scenario is clearly difficult to manage and very stressful. It is not possible to indicate a specific manualised intervention or strategy to deal with such a complex scenario. Mentalisation-based therapy offers some possible approaches that can help to de-escalate and contain such situations. Once again the goal is to re-establish mentalising on behalf of the patient which eventually facilitates their ability to appreciate the impossible demands they have placed on the clinician.

A mentalising approach would be to return to the most basic empathic stance and validate the patient's experience and distress. The idea is that the therapist has to acknowledge their role in precipitating the crisis, regardless of how extreme or irrational the patient's views or assumptions are. Only once this has occurred in a mentalising way, can the patient re-engage the clinician positively.

This can be incredibly difficult as the natural response is likely to be defensive, the clinician having genuinely had no intention at all to offend or upset. Moreover, the clinician's action even had the patient's interest at heart (not wanting to miss Michael's mum). The risk here is to further provoke and escalate the situation by adopting a polar, and ultimately entrenched, position in relation to the patient. This could be disastrous as the patient feels more and more undermined and angry.

Key question/intervention

Validate the patient's experience

Rewind to the moment before the break in mentalisation (your subjective continuity)

Explore the acute emotional context by identifying and naming the momentary affective state (feelings) between patient and clinician

Acknowledge your part in contributing to the break in mentalising

Attempt to mentalise the current emotional context (this could be done by offering an alternative perspective that provides an insight into the mind of another, but is only likely to work if the previous step was successful).

In general the type of mentalising intervention implemented can be seen as inversely related to the current level of emotional intensity. When someone is emotionally overwhelmed, it is most helpful to go back to support and empathy.

Summary

The mentalising stance is a helpful basis for all interactions between clinicians and young people. A mentalising intervention is most likely to be indicated if the clinician feels the young person struggles to mentalise and generally presents with marked 'borderline' characteristics. The TA diagram can provide a good focus for a specific mentalising intervention. Efforts to restore mentalisation can be very helpful at any time in the assessment process, especially in a moment of crisis during the assessment itself. The mentalising therapy described in this chapter is a simple and limited outline of what mentalisation-based therapy for borderline personality disorder entails and readers are encouraged to refer to more comprehensive texts to deepen their understanding of this approach.

Acknowledgement

Many of the concepts and examples in this chapter that relate to mentalisation and MBT are reproduced with the kind permission of Dr A. Bateman.

Reference

1.   Bateman A, Fonagy P. 8-year follow-up of patients treated for borderline personality disorder: mentalization-based treatment versus treatment as usual. *Am J Psychiatry* 2008;165:631–8.

CHAPTER 21

EMOTIONAL REGULATION AND DISTRESS TOLERANCE: PSYCHOLOGICAL FIRST AID

Dennis Ougrin

Introduction

At the time of writing, self-harm is understood as being primarily a manifestation of emotional dysregulation. Most of the previous chapters of this manual describe techniques that aim, to varying degrees, at developing young people's capacity for emotional regulation. Here we will review further techniques that clinicians might find useful when faced with a distressed young person. They are based primarily on the skills development programme of dialectical behaviour therapy (DBT).

Dialectical behaviour therapy was developed for the treatment of females with borderline personality disorder[1,2] and has since been modified for adolescents who self-harm.[3] The fundamental principle of DBT is derived from a dialectical approach to patients, on one hand accepting and understanding, on the other hand challenging and emphasising change. Dialectical behaviour therapy is a long-term treatment that could last several years. It comprises group sessions as well as individual sessions and telephone support.

A DBT programme has several phases:

1. decreasing life-threatening behaviours
2. decreasing therapy-interfering behaviours
3. decreasing quality-of-life interfering behaviours
4. increasing behavioural skills.

Throughout the treatment adolescents are taught 'replacement skills', categorised as follows:

1. core mindfulness
2. distress tolerance
3. interpersonal effectiveness
4. emotional regulation.

Unlike the adult version of DBT, DBT-A is shorter, involves more fun activities, uses modified language in handouts and involves families in therapeutic contact.

The techniques described below are based on the skills used in DBT; however, very similar techniques are used in mindfulness-based cognitive–behavioural therapy[4] and eye movement desensitisation and reprocessing (EMDR).[5]

Readers will find several exercises designed to improve emotional regulation and distress tolerance. These exercises are easy to learn and easy to practice. Some young people may find it useful to record the exercises; for example, using their mobile phones. The exercises should be done in a warm, quiet room that is adequately lit. Specific instructions for young people are in italics.

Breathing exercises

Basic breathing

1. I'd like to show you an exercise that some people find useful when they are stressed and it helps them relax. How does that sound? OK, please get comfortable in your chair. If you like, close your eyes or just look at the floor. (You need to make sure that the young person is sitting upright, without hunching over or crossing arms – the chest movements should be as free as possible.)

2. Scan your body from toes to head for any signs of tension, and just notice it. (Allow the young person a few seconds to do that.)

3. Now focus on your breathing. Notice how air enters your lungs and leaves your body. (You should ideally participate in the exercise and model the behaviour required.)

4. Let's take a deep breath together. Notice the sensation of coldness around the nose as you breathe in (pause). Follow the breath into the back of your mouth. Notice your lungs and chest expanding (pause). Now follow your breath all the way down to your belly. Hold your breath in for a second and than let it go slowly through your nose (pause). Follow your breath all the way out from your belly, through your lungs and chest, to the back of your mouth and nose. Notice the warmth around your nose as you breathe out.

5. OK, let's take another deep breath, notice, hold, let go.

6. One more time, inhale slowly and fully. Hold it for a second, and let go. Notice how with each breath your body becomes more relaxed and tension is leaving your body.

7. Now, let's continue breathing in this way for another minute or two. (Allow the young person to practice breathing for 1 to 2 minutes in silence.)

8. When you feel ready, open your eyes or look up again.

9. How was that? Did you notice any new sensations while you were breathing? How do you feel now?

    If the young person reports relaxing feelings, finish the exercise with this instruction:

10. You have done very well. Relaxing your breathing is a skill. It could be practiced just like any other skill and you could get better at it. Some people find it useful to practice deep breathing regularly, for say three minutes every day when they have a quiet time. You could then use deep breathing at times of distress or in your bed while trying to fall asleep or even on the bus or on a train.

Breathing with self-instruction

1. I'd like to show you an exercise that some people find useful when they are stressed and it helps them relax. How does that sound? OK, please get comfortable in your chair. If you like, close your eyes or just look at the floor. (You need to make sure that the young person is sitting upright, without hunching over or crossing arms – the chest movements should be as free as possible.)

2. Scan your body from toes to head for any signs of tension, and just notice it. (Allow the young person a few seconds to do this.)

3. Now focus on your breathing. Notice how air enters your lungs and leaves your body.

    (You should ideally participate in the exercise and model the behaviour required.)

4. Let's take a deep breath together. Notice the sensation of coldness around the nose as you breathe in (pause). Follow the breath into the back of your mouth. Notice your lungs and chest expanding (pause). Now follow your breath all the way down to your belly. Hold your breath in for a second and than let it go slowly through your nose (pause). Follow your breath all the way out from your belly, through your lungs and chest, to the back of your mouth and nose. Notice the warmth around your nose as you breathe out.

5. OK, let's take another deep breath, notice, hold, let go.

6. One more time, inhale slowly and fully. Hold your breath for a second, and let go.

7. Now the next time you breathe out, say slowly in your mind 'My head and neck are relaxed'. As you do it, notice how all the muscles in your head and your neck are relaxing. Let's take the next deep breath in together, hold it and let go. Continue breathing deeply and slowly in and out. Check for any tension in your head and neck, and let go.

    (Allow the young person to take two or three more breaths.)

8. The next time you breathe out, say slowly in your mind 'My chest my stomach and my back are relaxed'. As you do it, notice how all the muscles in your chest your stomach and your back are relaxing. Let's take the next deep breath in together, hold it and let go. Continue breathing deeply and slowly in and out. Check for any tension in your chest, your stomach and your back, and let go. (Allow the young person to take two or three more breaths.)

9. The next time you breathe out, say slowly in your mind 'My arms and my hands are relaxed'. As you do it, notice how all the muscles in your arms and your hands are relaxing. Let's take the next deep breath in together, hold it and let go. Continue breathing deeply and slowly in and out. Check for any tension in your arms and your hands, and let go.

   (Allow the young person to take two or three more breaths.)

10. The next time you breathe out, say slowly in your mind 'My legs and my feet are relaxed'. As you do it, notice how all the muscles in your legs and your feet are relaxing. Let's take the next deep breath in together, hold it and let go. Continue breathing deeply and slowly in and out. Check for any tension in your legs and your feet, and let go.

    (Allow the young person to take two or three more breaths.)

11. Now take another deep breath and the next time you breathe out, say slowly in your mind 'And now the whole of my body is relaxed'. As you do it, scan your body from head to toe and notice how all the muscles in your body are relaxing. Notice a wave of relaxation going all the way from head to toes. Let's take the next deep breath in together, hold it and let go. Continue breathing deeply and slowly in and out. Check for any tension in your legs and your feet, and let go.

12. Now, let's continue breathing in this way for another minute or two.

    (Allow the young person to practice breathing for 1–2 minutes in silence.)

13. When you feel ready, open your eyes or look up again.

14. How was that? Did you notice any new sensations while you were breathing? How do you feel now?

If the young person reports relaxing feelings, you could say

15. You have done very well. Muscle relaxation is a skill. It could be practised just like any other skill and you could get better at it. Some people find it useful to practice muscle relaxation regularly, for say three minutes every day when they have a quiet time. You could then use muscle relaxation at times of distress or in your bed while trying to fall asleep or even on the bus or on a train.

Below three modifications of the above exercises are described. The format is the same and the exercises should be finished with an encouragement to practise the skill.

Breathing with tension relaxation

If the young person reports that they still feel tension in their muscles, ask them to repeat the breathing exercise. Instead of relaxing the muscles, go over each muscle group, ask the young person to tense them hard and then relax them fully.

Breathing with hand over stomach

If breathing does not appear to be deep and slow, you might ask the young person to put a hand over their stomach and notice how it moves with each deep breath.

Breathing with elements of mindfulness

Start the exercise in the same way as you did breathing with self-instruction. When the young person is fully relaxed say:

1. Now observe any thoughts, ideas, feelings or images that enter your mind. Don't fight with them, don't try to push them away. Just observe.
   (Allow the young person to do this for a few seconds, then say:)
2. Just observe. Imagine that your thoughts (ideas feelings or images) are clouds in the sky, observe how they come, stay for a while and than go away.
   (Alternatively say:)
   Imagine that your thoughts (ideas feelings or images) are hot air balloons, you take them, hold them and then let go of them. Notice how the wind takes them away and they disappear.
   (Or:)
   Imagine your thoughts (ideas feelings or images) are on a conveyor belt, they appear, you see them for a while and then they disappear again.
   (Or:)
   Observe your thoughts (ideas feelings or images) as if you were watching them on a cinema screen. Take a seat in the audience and watch them play out.
3. It is inevitable that we will get caught up with the thoughts (ideas, feelings or images) over and over again. It is not a failure, just an opportunity to step back and watch the thoughts (ideas, feelings or images) play out again.

Finish the exercise as above.

Special place exercises

These exercises will be specific to each young person's experience and should describe a place or event (or both) that have a special meaning for the young person and are associated with positive emotions. Some young people may not be able to recall any event or place like that. If this is the case, you may try to get the young person to imagine a place or event like that in the future. All special places and events should be described in great detail. The descriptions should include as many of the five senses as possible.

1. I'd like you to remember a time when you felt especially good, safe or happy, like a holiday or a party, or a trip to the mountains.
   (Or:)
   I'd like you to imagine a place where you could feel especially good, safe or happy.
   (Or:)
   I'd like you to remember a time when you felt especially excited or had a sense of achievement.
   (Or:)
   I'd like you to remember a time when you were especially helpful or kind to other people.
2. Can you imagine yourself being there now? I'd like you to describe to me where you are. What can you see? Are there other people there? Are there any objects? What colour are they? Is there any movement?
3. Now please tell me if you can hear any sounds? Are they loud or quiet?
4. Can you feel or touch anything? What is under your feet? Can you feel the texture of the objects around you? What is it like?
5. Do you sense any smells? What are they like?
6. Is there anything you can taste? What is the taste like?
7. Stay in that place for a minute and enjoy any pleasant feelings or sensations in your body. Where can you feel them?
8. Now tell me what word or phrase would go best with this special place?
   (Allow the young person to ponder for a minute. If nothing is reported, you could say: 'Some people find that words like 'peace', 'calm', 'happiness' go well with their special places'.)
9. Keep this word and your special place together in your mind. Notice the pleasant feelings you have in your body as you hold the image and the word in your mind.
10. How was that? Did you notice any new sensations while you were breathing? How do you feel now? (If the young person responds positively to the experience.)
11. You have done very well. Using the special place exercise is a skill. It could be practised just like any other skill and you could get better at it. Some people find it useful to practise the special place exercise regularly, for say three minutes every day when they have a quiet time. You could then use the special place exercise at times of distress or in your bed while trying to fall asleep or even on the bus or on a train.

Observing exercises

Observing exercises could be practised in any environment. For these exercises to be effective the young person needs to be able to focus on their surroundings and report their experiences in detail. The descriptions could be based on any of the senses but in practise listening to sounds seems the most beneficial.

Listening to the sounds

1. I'd like to show you an exercise that some people find useful when they are stressed and it helps them relax. How does that sound? OK, please get comfortable in your chair. You could close your eyes or just look down at the floor.
2. Gradually become aware of the sounds you can hear in the room without judging them.
3. Label each sound in the room slowly as if you were tuning in to it like a microphone. Notice the pitch of the sound, the loudness, the rhythm and then let it go.
   (Allow the young person to do this for a few minutes.)
4. Now move your attention to the sounds outside of this room slowly as if you were tuning in to each of them like a microphone. Notice the pitch of the sound, the loudness, the rhythm and then let it go.
   (Allow the young person to continue for a few minutes.)
4. How was that? Did you notice any new sensations while you were doing the exercise? How do you feel now? (If the young person responds positively to the experience.)
5. You have done very well. Using the listening to the sounds exercise is a skill. It could be practised just like any other skill and you could get better at it. Some people find it useful to practise the listening to the sounds exercise regularly, for say three minutes every day when they have a quiet time. You could then use a listening to the sounds exercise at times of distress or in your bed while trying to fall asleep or even on the bus or on a train.

Observing exercises could in theory be done using all five senses as is clear from the exercise below.

Observing a raisin

A variation on this exercise could include a small food object, like a raisin, that the young person might hold on their hand. You could ask the young person to start by approaching the raisin as if they have never seen one before. Observe the shape, depth and texture of a raisin; then feel it with their fingers; examine its texture and unevenness; then place it in their mouth and notice salivation, texture and weight.

Then the young person should start to chew on it, noticing changes in taste, shape and texture. Finally the young person may observe how the raisin travels from their mouth into their stomach.

Clinical example

Gabby is a 17-year-old Portuguese British young lady who lives with her mother, step-father and three step-siblings and attends a college. She was referred by her GP with concerns regarding her mood and self-harm.

Gabby started self-harming at the age of 13 years. She was initially cutting her arms and then started cutting her chest and thighs. At the time of presentation she was cutting about twice a week with a clean razor. The main precipitants for her cutting were interpersonal conflicts, feeling rejected and left out by her family and experiencing thoughts of being fat, unattractive and lonely. This led to a mixture of anger, low mood and worry, as well as feeling as if she was 'unreal'. Cutting appeared to regulate these emotions in the short term but in the long term it had negative consequences, primarily leading to social rejection and being left out by her friends as well as feeling incompetent for not being able to regulate her emotions. During self-harm Gabby rarely felt pain (Figure 21.1).

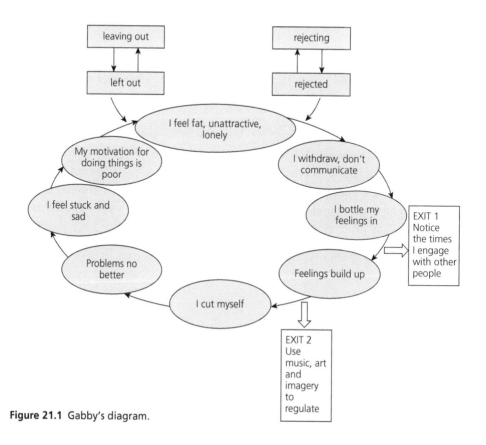

Figure 21.1 Gabby's diagram.

During the session, Gabby engaged well with therapeutic assessment, generating a diagram and suggesting two possible exits. When discussing her latest episode of self-harm, however, she became very upset. She also reported a feeling of tension in her body and she started sucking her thumb. The following exercise was undertaken.

T: Gabby?

G: (no response)

T: Gabby? (firmer, yet gently)

G: (made eye contact)

T: Gabby, it seems you are going through a difficult time right now

G: Yeah

T: I'd like to show you an exercise that many young people find useful when they feel bad. Is that OK?

G: um-hum

T: OK. Please sit up in the chair comfortably. Are you comfortable now?

G: Not really

T: Perhaps you may find it more comfortable to sit like this (shows a more open posture). Good. Could I ask you, if you have been on a holiday or a picnic or a trip to a forest?

G: Yeah

T: Right, can you remember the best one of those, the one you enjoyed most?

G: Yeah, last year we went to Madeira

T: That is great, was that the best holiday you have had?

G: (nod)

T: Could you tell me a little about that holiday, who did you go with, what did you do, that kind of thing?

G: It was just a good holiday. I spent lots of time with my mum and it was really great.

T: What did you enjoy most about it?

G: Shopping

T: I see; where did you do it?

G: A big shop in Santa Quitéria

T: What did you buy there?

G: I can't remember

T: OK, and what did you enjoy most?

G: Microlândia

T: What is that?

G: It's like a play area. We played bowling with my mum and I won

T: Right, can I ask you to imagine you are there now (pause). Are you there?

G: Kind of

T: Can you tell me what is going on?

G: We are playing

T: Could you get to the moment that is the most enjoyable?

G: Yeah

T: What is it?

G: I just won!

T: OK, please stay with that image. Tell me what do you see?

G: I can see the monitors and the other families, some small kids and my mum and …

T: The two of you?

G: Yeah

T: Anything else?

G: Yeah, the balls and the alley

T: Did you have a favourite ball?

G: Not really

T: OK, can you hear anything?

G: Yeah, there was some music, I can't remember it, but I can hear it

T: Any other noises?

G: People talking, my mum saying 'well done!'

T: In Portuguese?

G: Yeah, of course

T: What is 'well done' in Portuguese?

G: 'Parabéns!'

T: I see (pause), can you feel anything?*

G: Yeah, I feel really good

T: Right, and are you touching anything?

G: No, not really

T: What about any smells or tastes?

G: I can smell my mum's perfume

T: (pause) OK. How are you feeling now?

G: Good, I mean better

T: Can you point where that feeling is in your body?

G: Here (points to her chest)

T: What is it like?

G: Kind of like good

T: OK, I'd like you to focus on that feeling and picture yourself in the bowling alley again. Are you there?

---

*Confusion commonly happens at this point. The therapist was trying to get Gabby to enhance the image by asking her what she was touching. Instead, Gabby reported how she was feeling.

G: yeah

T: What word or phrase would go best with that image?

G: Parabéns!

T: Right. I'd like you to keep the image in your mind, feel the feeling in your body and repeat 'Parabéns!' in your mind

G: OK.

This exercise was followed by an experiment whereby Gabby remembered an upsetting event, but this time she was instructed to bring the image up and say 'Parabéns!' in her head. She was then invited to comment on the way her feelings changed and what she learned from the experiment.

Understanding Letter

Hi Gabby

Thank you very much for sharing your history with me and for helping me make sense of what has been going on in your life.

Please have a look at the diagram we made together – does it still look OK?

The two boxes at the top of the diagram are labelled 'rejecting'–'rejected', 'leaving out'–'left out'. When you find yourself 'rejected' and 'left out', you feel a mixture of sadness, loneliness and anger and you could have unhelpful thoughts about yourself. Although these thoughts are neither true nor helpful and do not have evidence to support them, they are important to be aware of as they start a cycle (see the diagram).

I will try to describe this and please forgive me if I did not record it exactly as you described it. You told me that when you feel bad and have the negative thoughts about yourself, it feels very difficult to share them with others. You described often bottling your thoughts and feelings in. This inevitably leads to a build-up of emotions and an 'explosion' – cutting. In the short term you feel better. The bad thoughts and feelings, however, don't really disappear and you feel stuck and sad. Sadness gets in the way of you feeling motivated to do things you are good at. This leads back to you having even more negative thoughts.

Did I get what you were saying right in this diagram? When we next meet, we could spend some time correcting any part of the diagram that doesn't seem right.

A cycle (see the diagram) can only work if all of its parts work together. If we can break one or two bits then it will not work any more.

I was especially impressed with the way you made the first steps towards breaking this cycle yourself. You discovered that withdrawing and not talking to anyone does not work and that making the first step to communicate with others feels good and makes your mood better.

Second, your mother suggested that at times when you feel overcome with emotions you can use music and art to express your feelings. This could be the second 'exit' from the cycle.

We then did a brief exercise looking at other ways you might manage difficult emotions. You remembered, in great detail, a time in Madeira when you were bowling with your mum and you won. You remembered what you saw, heard and smelled that day and you also remembered 'Parabéns!' the expression that went well with the whole experience. We then did another exercise where you managed to challenge a negative feeling by saying 'Parabéns!' and remembered the image again.

It may be helpful to notice the times when you could manage difficult feelings by practising this exercise. When we meet again next Thursday at 4 pm, we could do some more thinking about how best to manage these feelings.

Thanks once again for your hard work today

With best regards,

Dennis

Summary

Exercises and skills directed at emotional regulation and distress tolerance are key skills of psychological first aid. Moreover, they might be useful in improving young people's experiences of the initial assessment and could also improve motivation for change and hope for the future. Not all therapists will have the opportunity to engage adolescents presenting with self-harm with coherent mindfulness-based treatment programmes, but using emotional regulation/distress tolerance exercises might inform any intervention. Many young people enjoy practising these skills and report a sense of mastery and pleasure as they improve.

References

1. Linehan MM, Armstrong HE, Suarez A, Allmon D, Heard HL. Cognitive-behavioral treatment of chronically parasuicidal borderline patients [see comment]. *Arch Gen Psychiatry* 1991;48(12):1060–4.
2. Linehan MM, Schmidt H, 3rd, Dimeff LA, *et al.* Dialectical behavior therapy for patients with borderline personality disorder and drug-dependence. *Am J Addict* 1999;8(4):279–92.
3. Rathus JH, Miller AL. Dialectical Behavior Therapy adapted for suicidal adolescents. *Suicide Life Threat Behav* 2002;32(2):146–57.
4. Kuyken W, Byford S, Taylor RS, *et al.* Mindfulness-based cognitive therapy to prevent relapse in recurrent depression. *J Consult Clin Psychol* 2008;76(6):966–78.
5. Ahmad A, Larsson B, Sundelin-Wahlsten V. EMDR treatment for children with PTSD: results of a randomized controlled trial. *Nord J Psychiatry* 2007;61(5):349–54.

Concluding remarks

We would like to finish with this short story. There was a little girl called Cinderella. She generally had a very bad time with her family and her friends were not what they could have been. One day she was really upset and her fairy godmother came along with a magical wand. But her magical wand could only make shoes. Cinderella was very grateful to her fairy godmother but she was quite angry as well. She told the fairy godmother: 'Thank you fairy godmother, I'm going to keep the shoes in my cupboard. But if your magic wand could create other things, I wouldn't mind having them too, otherwise I am not going to be able to go to the royal ball'. The fairy godmother scratched her head: 'I could learn how to make other things with my magical wand, but I will need someone to help me', she said. So, she went on the internet and found lots of other fairies who each learned how to make different things with their wands. They all got together and taught each other and had monthly supervision sessions. Then the fairy godmother came back to Cinderella's house. Unfortunately, she was nowhere to be found. While the fairy godmother was studying her magic, Cinderella went to university, found her Prince Charming, sat exams at the Institute of Management Accountancy and became financial director of a FTSE 100 company. 'Don't fool yourself, fairy godmother', she said 'I could do well with your magic, but with my own determination I can do even better. In the end I realised it wasn't you who had to do something different'.

Index

Numbers in **bold** type indicate Tables; those in *italics* indicate Figures.